Loss and Trauma in the COVID-19 Era

The COVID pandemic (including the COVID and its complications) killed around 7 million people, according to the World Health Organization (WHO). This unique book includes 19 chapters by an international cast of authors, addressing aspects of loss and trauma connected to the virus, including COVID and posttraumatic stress, COVID and love, COVID and bereaved families, COVID and ageism, and COVID and world orderliness.

A central theme in this volume is the attempt by scholars and practitioners to provide hope in the midst of a sense of global darkness that accompanied the burgeoning spread of the virus in 2020. It explores a range of COVID-related topics that bear on loss and trauma. The book is a valuable read for scholars and students researching on and dealing with trauma, as well as for practitioners working with clients who have COVID-related problems. The book will also benefit general readers interested in impacts of the pandemic on loss and trauma.

The chapters in this book were originally published as two special issues in *Journal of Loss and Trauma.*

John H. Harvey is Professor Emeritus of Psychology at the University of Iowa, USA. His research and writing foci have been on loss and trauma and interpersonal relationships. He is the founding Editor of the *Journal of Loss and Trauma.*

Loss and Trauma in the COVID-19 Era

Edited by
John H. Harvey

Routledge
Taylor & Francis Group
LONDON AND NEW YORK

First published 2024
by Routledge
4 Park Square, Milton Park, Abingdon, Oxon OX14 4RN

and by Routledge
605 Third Avenue, New York, NY 10158

Routledge is an imprint of the Taylor & Francis Group, an informa business

British Library Cataloguing in Publication Data
A catalogue record for this book is available from the British Library

ISBN13: 978-1-032-64785-2 (hbk)
ISBN13: 978-1-032-64786-9 (pbk)
ISBN13: 978-1-032-64787-6 (ebk)

DOI: 10.4324/9781032647876

Typeset in Minion Pro
by Newgen Publishing UK

Publisher's Note
The publisher accepts responsibility for any inconsistencies that may have arisen during the conversion of this book from journal articles to book chapters, namely the inclusion of journal terminology.

Contents

Citation Information

The chapters in this book were originally published in the *Journal of Loss and Trauma*, volume 25, issues 6–7 and 8 (2020). When citing this material, please use the original page numbering for each article, as follows:

Introduction

JLT and the Coronavirus
John H. Harvey
Journal of Loss and Trauma, volume 25, issue 6–7 (2020), pp. 501–502

Chapter 1

Coronavirus Disease (COVID-19) and Traumatic Stress: Probable Risk Factors and Correlates of Posttraumatic Stress Disorder
Güler Boyraz and Dominique N. Legros
Journal of Loss and Trauma, volume 25, issue 6–7 (2020), pp. 503–522

Chapter 2

Managing COVID-19 in a Large Urban Research-Intensive University
Cheryl Regehr and Vivek Goel
Journal of Loss and Trauma, volume 25, issue 6–7 (2020), pp. 523–539

Chapter 3

Romantic Love in the Age of COVID-19
Susan S. Hendrick and Clyde Hendrick
Journal of Loss and Trauma, volume 25, issue 6–7 (2020), pp. 540–543

Chapter 4

Reaction to the COVID-19 Pandemic: The Influence of Meaning in Life, Life Satisfaction, and Assumptions on World Orderliness and Positivity
Jerzy Trzebiński, Maciej Cabański, and Jolanta Zuzanna Czarnecka
Journal of Loss and Trauma, volume 25, issue 6–7 (2020), pp. 544–557

Chapter 5

Longing for a Familiar Way of Going Forward
Peter Joseph Gloviczki
Journal of Loss and Trauma, volume 25, issue 6–7 (2020), pp. 558–559

Chapter 6
The COVID-19 Pandemic Crisis: The Loss and Trauma Event of Our Time
Eric D. Miller
Journal of Loss and Trauma, volume 25, issue 6–7 (2020), pp. 560–572

Chapter 7
Philippine Teachers' Practices to Deal with Anxiety amid COVID-19
Karen Joy B. Talidong and Cathy Mae D. Toquero
Journal of Loss and Trauma, volume 25, issue 6–7 (2020), pp. 573–579

Chapter 8
Mental Health and Its Influencing Factors among Self-Isolating Ordinary Citizens during the Beginning Epidemic of COVID-19
Yuqing Zhao, Yuanyuan An, Xing Tan, and Xiaohui Li
Journal of Loss and Trauma, volume 25, issue 6–7 (2020), pp. 580–593

Chapter 9
A Glimpse of University Students' Family Life Amidst the COVID-19 Virus
Haimin Pan
Journal of Loss and Trauma, volume 25, issue 6–7 (2020), pp. 594–597

Chapter 10
Stranded College Students amid Corona Virus Disease 2019 Pandemic: An Existential Phenomenology
Michael B. Cahapay
Journal of Loss and Trauma, volume 25, issue 6–7 (2020), pp. 598–604

Chapter 11
A Researcher and Survivor of the Holocaust Connect and Make Meaning during the COVID-19 Pandemic
Carolyn Ellis and Jerry Rawicki
Journal of Loss and Trauma, volume 25, issue 6–7 (2020), pp. 605–622

Chapter 12
Impact of COVID-19 on Athletes and Coaches, and Their Values in Japan: Repercussions of Postponing the Tokyo 2020 Olympic and Paralympic Games
Kanako Taku and Hirokazu Arai
Journal of Loss and Trauma, volume 25, issue 8 (2020), pp. 623–630

Chapter 13
Defining a 'Risk Group' and Ageism in the Era of COVID-19
Atiqur Rahman and Yasmin Jahan
Journal of Loss and Trauma, volume 25, issue 8 (2020), pp. 631–634

Chapter 14

Knowledge, Attitudes, Anxiety, and Coping Strategies of Students during COVID-19 Pandemic
Erick T. Baloran
Journal of Loss and Trauma, volume 25, issue 8 (2020), pp. 635–642

Chapter 15

Together for Hope and Resilience: A Humanistic Experience by the Vulnerability, Trauma, Resilience and Culture Lab Members during the COVID-19 Pandemic
Jude Mary Cénat, Pari-Gole Noorishad, Camille Blais-Rochette, Sara-Emilie McIntee, Joana N. Mukunzi, Wina Paul Darius, Cathy Broussard, Catherine Morse, Gloria Ukwu, Emmanuelle Auguste, and Kerry Menelas
Journal of Loss and Trauma, volume 25, issue 8 (2020), pp. 643–648

Chapter 16

The Impact of Social Uncertainty, Protests, and COVID-19 on Hong Kong Teachers
Kevin M. Wong and Benjamin Luke Moorhouse
Journal of Loss and Trauma, volume 25, issue 8 (2020), pp. 649–655

Chapter 17

The Effects of Incriminating COVID-19 News on the Returning Indonesians' Anxiety
Mahir Pradana, Syahputra Syahputra, Aditya Wardhana, Budi Rustandi Kartawinata, and Candra Wijayangka
Journal of Loss and Trauma, volume 25, issue 8 (2020), pp. 656–661

Chapter 18

COVID-19: An Australian Perspective
Jane Shakespeare-Finch, Holly Bowen-Salter, Miranda Cashin, Amalia Badawi, Ruth Wells, Simon Rosenbaum, and Zachary Steel
Journal of Loss and Trauma, volume 25, issue 8 (2020), pp. 662–672

Chapter 19

The Future That Awaits Us
Peter Joseph Gloviczki
Journal of Loss and Trauma, volume 25, issue 8 (2020), pp. 673–674

Notes on Contributors

Yuanyuan An, School of Psychology, Nanjing Normal University, Nanjing, P. R. China.

Hirokazu Arai, Department of Psychology, Faculty of Letters, Hosei University, Tokyo, Japan.

Emmanuelle Auguste, School of Psychology, University of Ottawa, Ottawa, Canada.

Amalia Badawi, Graduate School of Health, University of Technology Sydney, Sydney, Australia.

Erick T. Baloran, College of Teacher Education, University of Mindanao – Bansalan College, Bansalan, Philippines.

Camille Blais-Rochette, School of Psychology, University of Ottawa, Ottawa, Canada.

Holly Bowen-Salter, Military and Emergency Services Health Australia, Australia.

Güler Boyraz, Department of Psychology, Pace University, New York City, New York, USA.

Cathy Broussard, School of Psychology, University of Ottawa, Ottawa, Canada.

Maciej Cabański, Faculty of Psychology, SWPS University, Warsaw, Poland.

Michael B. Cahapay, College of Education, Mindanao State University, General Santos City, Philippines.

Miranda Cashin, Clinical Psychology Unit, University of Sydney, Sydney, Australia.

Jude Mary Cénat, School of Psychology, University of Ottawa, Ottawa, Canada.

Jolanta Zuzanna Czarnecka, Faculty of Psychology, SWPS University, Warsaw, Poland.

Wina Paul Darius, School of Psychology, University of Ottawa, Ottawa, Canada.

Carolyn Ellis, Department of Communication, University of South Florida, Tampa, Florida, USA.

Peter Joseph Gloviczki, Department of Broadcasting and Journalism, Western Illinois University, Macomb, Illinois, USA.

Vivek Goel, University of Waterloo, Waterloo, Canada.

John H. Harvey, Department of Psychological & Brain Sciences, University of Iowa, Iowa City, Iowa, USA.

Clyde Hendrick, Department of Psychological Sciences, Texas Tech University, Lubbock, Texas, USA.

Susan S. Hendrick, Department of Psychological Sciences, Texas Tech University, Lubbock, Texas, USA.

Yasmin Jahan, London School of Hygiene and Tropical Medicine, London, UK.

Budi Rustandi Kartawinata, Department of Business Administration, Telkom University, Bandung, Indonesia.

Dominique N. Legros, Department of Psychology, Pace University, New York City, New York, USA.

Xiaohui Li, School of Family and Consumer Sciences, Northern Illinois University, DeKalb, Illinois, USA.

Sara-Emilie McIntee, School of Psychology, University of Ottawa, Ottawa, Canada.

Kerry Menelas, School of Psychology, University of Ottawa, Ottawa, Canada.

Eric D. Miller, Psychology Department, Kent State University, East Liverpool, Ohio, USA.

Benjamin Luke Moorhouse, Faculty of Education, Hong Kong Baptist University, Hong Kong, P. R. China.

Catherine Morse, School of Psychology, University of Ottawa, Ottawa, Canada.

Joana N. Mukunzi, School of Psychology, University of Ottawa, Ottawa, Canada.

Pari-Gole Noorishad, School of Psychology, University of Ottawa, Ottawa, Canada.

Haimin Pan, Xiamen University, Fujian, P. R. China.

Mahir Pradana, Department of Business Administration, Telkom University, Bandung, Indonesia.

Atiqur Rahman, Department of Culture and Society, Division Ageing and Social Change, Linköping University, Sweden.

Jerry Rawicki, Independent Scholar, St. Petersburg, Florida, USA.

Cheryl Regehr, Factor-Inwentash Faculty of Social Work, University of Toronto, Toronto, Canada.

Simon Rosenbaum, School of Psychiatry, University of New South Wales, Sydney, Australia.

Jane Shakespeare-Finch, Faculty of Health, School of Psychology & Counselling, Queensland University of Technology, Brisbane, Australia.

Zachary Steel, School of Psychiatry, University of New South Wales, Sydney, Australia.

Syahputra Syahputra, Department of Business Administration, Telkom University, Bandung, Indonesia.

Kanako Taku, Department of Psychology, Oakland University, Rochester, Michigan, USA.

Karen Joy B. Talidong, School of Education, Shaanxi Normal University, Xi'an, P. R. China.

Xing Tan, School of Psychology, South China Normal University, Guangzhou, Guangdong, P. R. China.

Cathy Mae D. Toquero, College of Education, Mindanao State University, General Santos City, Philippines.

Jerzy Trzebiński, Faculty of Psychology, SWPS University, Warsaw, Poland.

Gloria Ukwu, School of Psychology, University of Ottawa, Ottawa, Canada.

Aditya Wardhana, Department of Business Administration, Telkom University, Bandung, Indonesia.

Ruth Wells, School of Psychiatry, University of New South Wales, Sydney, Australia.

Candra Wijayangka, Department of Business Administration, Telkom University, Bandung, Indonesia.

Kevin M. Wong, Graduate School of Education and Psychology, Pepperdine University, Los Angeles, California, USA.

Yuqing Zhao, School of Psychology, Nanjing Normal University, Nanjing, P. R. China.

Introduction: JLT and the Coronavirus

Lifton (1996) said that we live on images. That is grimly true with the worldwide encounter with the Coronavirus that has begun to occupy our thoughts, feelings, and actions in early 2020. JLT has a role to play in this preoccupation. JLT was created in 1995 to address the topic of loss, broadly construed, and including trauma. It was asserted that loss is a pervasive experience in all human lives, and that JLT would serve as an outlet for scholarship addressing the many types and facets of loss (Harvey, 1996). Hopefully, the journal has fulfilled, and is fulfilling, that mission to some significant degree.

With the pandemic of the Coronavirus, loss is becoming a more salient international experience, just as other viruses and other events such as world wars did in different times. Collectively, we experience the feeling of loss of health, of safety and security, of economic well-being, of social interaction, of travel, of entertainment, of life itself, and much more.

This Editorial is meant to encourage a type of hope that scholars can provide via their writing and research. Hope is the bottom-line in this endeavor. What types of scholarship does the Editorial Board at JLT encourage in this situation? One straightforward type of work would be surveys and interviews especially with the elderly, but also with persons in various age ranges, about their fears, hopes, and attempts to deal with the Virus; such an inquiry with the elderly would be especially important given the Virus' apparent predominance in older persons. Similarly, surveys and interviews with medical personnel and first responders who must surrender a significant amount of safety and security in order to help the sick and dying. Counselors and mental health workers also have important feelings to report from their work in helping people deal with their fears about the Virus. Other groups who likely would have unique and informative experiences to report are athletes and entertainers, whose seasons, travels, and economic opportunities may have been cut short by the Virus.

Ironically, one group that deserves scrutiny in this long list are scholars and teachers themselves. With universities and schools suspending operations for lengthy periods of time, the very mission and livelihood of the teacher/scholar are in peril. Even research involving in-person interviewing of individuals is being restricted.

The above foci are particularly open to case studies and autoethnography that have formed a significant segment of JLT articles since its inception. The concept of imagery suggests a type of work that would survey media reports and opinion-editorial pieces about the Virus, and possibly how people react to these presentations. For example, it was reported that a newspaper in a moderate-sized Italian town had increased its obituary section from a customary one page to 14 pages as the Virus raged in mid-March. How do people react to such news? We know that cynicism has grown in the United States, as the severity of the Virus was not well-recognized and -addressed in the early weeks of its spread to the United States. Research could be done to better understand that cynicism and its effects in different countries, or internationally. The same type of study could be done for other prominent activities emerging in this context (e.g., bonding and greater faith; acts of giving and humanitarianism) reported in the media and by individuals.

Finally, JLT is open to analyses without typical data, whether quantitative or qualitative, that explore the nature of loss associated with the Virus. In sum, JLT is open for business to do its part in encouraging a greater sense of hope in the "age of the Coronavirus."

References

Harvey, J. H. (1996). Editorial and commentary: On the creation of the. *Journal of Personal and Interpersonal Loss. (JLT)*, *1*(1), iii–ii9. https://doi.org/10.1080/15325029608415453

Lifton, R. J. (1996). *The broken connection*. American Psychiatric Press.

John H. Harvey

Coronavirus Disease (COVID-19) and Traumatic Stress: Probable Risk Factors and Correlates of Posttraumatic Stress Disorder

Güler Boyraz and Dominique N. Legros

ABSTRACT
The Coronavirus Disease (COVID-19) outbreak, which first began in December 2019 in China, has since become a global health crisis with vast and devastating consequences for individuals and societies. Both earlier research and recent findings suggest that infectious disease epidemics and pandemics can be highly traumatic experiences for some individuals and lead to posttraumatic stress disorder (PTSD) and chronic psychological distress. Mental health risks associated with COVID-19 have yet to be systematically studied; however, the emerging literature on COVID-19, as well as previous studies on infectious disease outbreaks provide insights into probable risk factors and correlates of PTSD. In this paper, we provide a brief review of these studies and discuss probable risk factors for PTSD and chronic psychological distress related to COVID-19.

Coronavirus Disease (COVID-19) is caused by a new and highly contagious coronavirus (severe acute respiratory syndrome coronavirus 2 [SARS-CoV-2]; World Health Organization, 2020a) that was first identified in December 2019 in Wuhan, China (World Health Organization, 2020b). On March 11, 2020, the Director-General of the World Health Organization described the COVID-19 outbreak as a pandemic, noting that 118,000 confirmed cases and 4291 deaths had been reported in 114 countries (World Health Organization, 2020c). Since then, COVID-19 has continued to spread rapidly across the world, leading to 213 countries or regions with reported cases, and over 200,000 reported deaths worldwide as of April 28, 2020 (World Health Organization, 2020d, 2020e).

As the number of infected persons and the death toll continue to mount across the world, so does the psychological and economic toll on individuals and societies. As of April 26, New York State is one of the most adversely affected regions in the world, with over 288,000 confirmed cases (New York State Department of Health, 2020b) and 16,966 confirmed deaths (New York State Department of Health, 2020a). A weekly survey conducted by the City University of New York (CUNY), which began on March 13, 2020, indicated that many New York residents have been experiencing various pandemic-related worries and stressors (e.g., a rising perceived threat of becoming infected, social isolation, job/financial loss, economic stressors including the inability to pay rent and fear of being evicted; CUNY Graduate School of Public Health and Health Policy, 2020a), many of which have been linked to increased posttraumatic stress and other mental health problems in previous literature (Bonanno et al., 2008; Wu et al., 2005; Yu et al., 2005). The fourth week's (April 3–5; $n = 1000$) results of this survey indicated that 43% of New York City (NYC) residents knew someone who had COVID-19 and approximately half of them (48%) rated their chance of becoming infected as "high" or "very high." The majority of the NYC residents (60%) who participated in this survey reported hopelessness about the future and many of them felt socially isolated (40%), anxious (44%), or depressed (35%) "at least half of the time" during the past week. In addition, 40% of the participants indicated that the major contributing factor to their distress is their concern about family members or loved ones getting sick (CUNY Graduate School of Public Health and Health Policy, 2020c).

Parallel to these findings, a recent survey of more than a thousand adults in China highlighted the psychological impact of COVID-19 (Wang et al., 2020). Wang et al. (2020) reported that three-quarters of the participants (75.2%) expressed concerns about their family members getting sick. In addition, more than half of the participants (53.8%) perceived the psychological impact of the COVID-19 outbreak as "moderate" or "severe" and a smaller percentage of the participants reported "moderate" to "severe" symptoms of anxiety (16.5%), depression (28.8%), and stress (8.1%).

Although fear, anxiety, and stress are common and natural reactions to a global health crisis that affects every domain of life and confronts individuals with the fragility of life, both earlier research (Hong et al., 2009; Lau et al., 2004; Mak et al., 2010) and recent findings (Liu et al., 2020; Sun et al., 2020) suggest that infectious disease epidemics and pandemics can be traumatic experiences for some people, and lead to posttraumatic stress disorder (PTSD) and chronic psychological symptoms. A recent study (Liu et al., 2020) examined the prevalence of COVID-19-specific PTSD symptoms in a sample of adults ($n = 285$) living in Wuhan and surrounding cities in China and reported that 7% of participants met the diagnostic criteria for PTSD. In addition, participants who live in Wuhan, one of the highly affected areas in the world, reported higher posttraumatic stress than those who live in surrounding areas (Liu et al., 2020).

Findings from earlier infectious disease literature also suggest that many individuals experience deteriorations in their well-being and some individuals develop PTSD after infectious disease outbreaks. For example, several studies (Bonanno et al., 2008; Lau et al., 2004; Mak et al., 2010; Wu et al., 2005; Yu et al., 2005) examined mental health outcomes associated with the severe acute respiratory syndrome (SARS; a viral respiratory condition that resembles COVID-19 in its clinical features; see Petrosillo et al., 2020) which was first identified in Asia in February 2003 and spread to more than 20 countries within a few months (Centers for Disease Control and Prevention, 2017). In one of these studies, Lau et al. (2004) examined Hong Kong residents' psychological responses to the SARS outbreak and reported that more than half of the residents felt helpless (65.4%), horrified (55.5%), or apprehensive (65.0%) due to SARS, and 48.4% reported that "their mental health had severely or moderately deteriorated because of the SARS epidemic" (p. 420). In addition, 13.3% of men and 18% of women reported elevated PTSD symptomatology and many participants reported increased stress (work stress, financial stress, or family stress), sleep problems, and increased frequency of smoking or alcohol use after the SARS epidemic (Lau et al., 2004).

While the COVID-19 pandemic bears some similarities to the SARS epidemic, it has been more widespread and has led to a greater number of hospitalizations and deaths worldwide. In addition, COVID-19 continues to spread rapidly across the world, affecting more people every day in various ways (e.g., financial losses, job loss, difficulty accessing vital supplies, increasing social isolation, uncertainties about the future); thus, mental health effects of the COVID-19 pandemic will be more widespread and may be more profound than those of the SARS epidemic. While some countries are currently less affected by COVID-19, residents of these countries may still experience anticipatory anxiety due to the rapid spread of the virus. Research suggests that anticipatory anxiety is a common experience during and after infectious disease outbreaks (Lau et al., 2004; Liao et al., 2014; Limcaoco et al., 2020). For example, following the SARS outbreak, many people in Hong Kong believed that SARS would return in the following months (Lau et al., 2004). Therefore, uncertainties about the future and feelings of anxiety and fear may continue to be prevalent even after COVID-19 is eradicated.

While infectious disease pandemics can be highly stressful for all individuals, research suggests that the psychological impact of these collective traumas may be more severe for some individuals due to certain risk factors, such as greater exposure to the disease (e.g., becoming infected, living in highly affected areas, knowing someone who has been infected; Jiang et al., 2020; Lee et al., 2006; Sun et al., 2020). In addition, some populations may be disproportionately affected by COVID-19 both in terms of the level of exposure, as well as the amount and type of stressors they experience.

Consequently, they may be at higher risk of developing PTSD and other mental health problems. Although mental health risk factors associated with COVID-19 have yet to be systematically studied, the emerging literature on COVID-19, as well as previous studies on infectious disease outbreaks provide insights into probable risk factors for PTSD and chronic psychological distress. In this paper, we provide a brief review of these studies and discuss probable risk factors for PTSD and chronic psychological dysfunction related to COVID-19.

Probable risk factors for PTSD and chronic psychological dysfunction

Level of exposure

The emerging literature on COVID-19 suggests that the prevalence of PTSD is higher among individuals who have greater exposure to COVID-19. Sun et al. (2020) collected survey data from a general sample of adults in mainland China ($n = 2091$) and found that 4.6% of the participants endorsed symptoms suggesting a probable PTSD diagnosis. However, the prevalence of probable PTSD was significantly higher (18.4%) in a subsample of participants with greater exposure to COVID-19 (i.e., participants with suspected or confirmed COVID-19 diagnoses and those who have had close contact with a person who had COVID-19). The authors reported that poor sleep quality, being a woman, and recent exposure to Wuhan city (e.g., living in or traveling to Wuhan) were associated with increased PTSD symptomatology. Similarly, another recent study indicated that greater exposure to COVID-19 (e.g., being a friend or family member of a health-care worker or a person infected with COVID-19; having friends or family members with a recent history of visiting Wuhan) was associated with moderate or severe PTSD symptomatology (Jiang et al., 2020).

Similar results have been reported in the SARS literature. For example, in a study conducted in Hong Kong (Lee et al., 2006), 14% of the middle-aged and older adults living in SARS-prevalent areas reported clinically significant levels of posttraumatic stress; whereas, the prevalence of elevated PTSD symptomatology was significantly lower among those who live in less affected areas (3%). Further, for those living in SARS-prevalent areas, older adults were more likely to report elevated PTSD symptomatology (20%) than middle-aged adults (5.9%). It is important to note that none of the participants in this study had relatives, close friends, significant others, or neighbors (in the same building) with a history of SARS. Therefore, living in highly affected areas can be an independent risk factor for PTSD—particularly among older adults—even if individuals and those who are close to them do not contract the disease.

Loss of a loved one

The prevalence of PTSD among individuals who have lost their loved ones due to COVID-19 has not been examined yet; however, previous literature suggests that the sudden and unexpected death of a loved one is a risk factor for several mental disorders, including PTSD, major depressive disorder, panic disorder, and alcohol use disorders (Keyes et al., 2014). Because COVID-19 is highly contagious, some people may experience multiple losses within their families or communities. In addition, considering the social, psychological, economic, and physical health consequences of COVID-19, many people may experience multiple forms of loss (e.g., loss of a loved one, loss of health, financial loss, job loss, loss of social connection, loss of security), which may complicate the grieving process and increase the likelihood of developing PTSD and chronic psychological distress. Further, COVID-19 has forced individuals to make significant adjustments in their lives, including funeral rituals and how individuals say goodbye to their loved ones. Previous research suggests that participation in funeral arrangements and feeling comforted by funeral rituals contribute positively to bereavement adjustment (Gamino et al., 2000). Given the critical role of funeral rituals in bereavement adjustment, individuals who are unable to hold a proper funeral for their loved ones due to COVID-19 may experience more intense and prolonged distress.

Hospitalization for COVID-19

While our knowledge of the psychological impact of COVID-19 on hospitalized COVID-19 patients and survivors is limited, a recent study conducted in China (Bo et al., 2020) indicated that the prevalence of PTSD can be staggeringly high among hospitalized COVID-19 patients. Bo et al. (2020) recruited 714 clinically stable COVID-19 patients from temporary quarantine hospitals located in Wuhan, China. Using the PTSD Checklist—Civilian Version (PCL-C; Weathers et al., 1993), the authors reported that 96.2% of the patients met the cutoff score for probable PTSD (i.e., a total score of 50 or higher on PCL-C), suggesting that almost all patients experienced clinically significant levels of posttraumatic stress. It is important to note, however, that the authors of this study used the PCL-C, which measures the symptoms of PTSD in relation to general stressors (rather than a specific stressful event); therefore, it is unknown whether participants of this study reported their symptoms in relation to COVID-19 or other stressful events they may have experienced in the past.

The long-term psychological effects of COVID-19 on hospitalized patients are currently unknown; however, based on previous studies with hospitalized survivors of SARS (Bonanno et al., 2008; Hong et al., 2009;

Lee et al., 2007; Mak et al., 2010), hospitalization for COVID-19 can be considered a foreseeable risk factor for PTSD and chronic psychological distress. Studies that examined the long-term psychological outcomes among SARS survivors indicated that these individuals experienced different challenges at different stages of their recovery (e.g., psychotic symptoms and fear for their lives and of infecting others during early stages of recovery; perceived stigmatization, distress, and decreased quality of life in later stages) and many of them experienced significant distress for months—even years—after hospitalization (for a review, see Gardner & Moallef, 2015). Bonanno et al. (2008) followed 997 SARS survivors from 6 to 18 months after their hospitalization in order to examine the psychological functioning trajectories of these individuals. While many participants in this study maintained high levels of psychological functioning throughout the study (35%) or demonstrated a pattern of psychological recovery over time (10%), 42% of the participants had low levels of psychological functioning at 6 months post-hospitalization and did not show improvements in their functioning over time. An additional 13% of the participants had high psychological functioning initially, but reported declines in their functioning over time (Bonanno et al., 2008).

Other studies indicated that a relatively large percentage of SARS survivors developed PTSD after hospitalization. For example, Mak et al. (2010) interviewed 90 Chinese adults who had been hospitalized for SARS approximately 30 months after the SARS outbreak and reported that slightly less than half of these participants (47.8%) developed PTSD sometime after the outbreak and 25.6% met the diagnostic criteria for PTSD at 30 months following the outbreak. Hong et al. (2009) collected longitudinal data from a sample of SARS survivors ($n = 68$) across five time-points (from 2 months to 46 months after being discharged from the hospital) and reported that 44.1% of the participants developed PTSD at some point during the study period. In another study, Kwek et al. (2006) reported that the prevalence of probable PTSD was 41.7% at three months post-hospital discharge among SARS survivors.

The PTSD prevalence rates reported for SARS survivors and COVID-19 patients are considerably higher than for individuals who are exposed to other potentially traumatic events, such as sexual assault, motor vehicle accidents, and other life-threatening events (for a review, see Bonanno, 2004). In addition, the prevalence of chronic psychological dysfunction among trauma-exposed populations tends to range from five to 10%; whereas, a considerably higher percentage of SARS survivors (42%) exhibited chronic psychological dysfunction (see Bonanno, 2004; Bonanno et al., 2008).

Taken together, being hospitalized for COVID-19 might be a significant risk factor for PTSD and chronic psychological dysfunction. This risk may be higher for individuals who develop more severe illness and/or for those who have additional risk factors. For example, preexisting chronic medical conditions, treatment-related complications (Mak et al., 2010), low social support, more epidemic related worries (e.g., fear of infecting others, feeling unsafe about oneself, worrying about family members' health, increased thoughts about death and dying), and poor physical functioning (Bonanno et al., 2008) were related to increased PTSD symptomatology or chronic psychological dysfunction among SARS survivors. Therefore, early detection of risk factors and early intervention may play a critical role in mitigating the effects of COVID-19 on psychological functioning for individuals who have been hospitalized for COVID-19.

Isolation and quarantine

While pandemic containment measures, such as travel restrictions, business closures, social distancing, and quarantine play a critical role in slowing down the spread of COVID-19, some of these protective measures have been linked to PTSD and other mental health problems (for a review, see Brooks et al., 2020; Hawryluck et al., 2004; Sprang & Silman, 2013). In a sample of Toronto residents who were placed in home- or work-quarantine during the SARS epidemic, Hawryluck et al. (2004) found that 28.9% of the participants reported elevated PTSD symptomatology and 31.2% reported depressive symptomatology after the quarantine period. In addition, lower household income and longer quarantine duration were associated with higher PTSD symptomatology (Hawryluck et al., 2004). In another study, the prevalence of probable PTSD was considerably higher among parents and children who were quarantined or isolated during infectious disease outbreaks (i.e., H1N1, SARS, or avian influenza outbreaks) than among parents and children who did not experience quarantine or isolation (Sprang & Silman, 2013). The results of this study also indicated the mean posttraumatic stress score of the quarantined or isolated children was four times higher than that of children who did not experience quarantine or isolation (Sprang & Silman, 2013).

These findings suggest that quarantine and isolation can be highly traumatic experiences for both children and adults. Other disease containment measures, such as travel restrictions and business closures will likely be highly stressful for many people, including individuals who lost their jobs due to business closures and those who are away from their home country and unable to return due to travel restrictions.

Social inequalities and related risk factors

Socially disadvantaged individuals, such as those with lower-income have been disproportionately affected during past infectious disease outbreaks (e.g., greater exposure to infectious diseases and higher mortality rates; Blumenshine et al., 2008; Mamelund, 2004; Quinn et al., 2011; Quinn & Kumar, 2014; Sydenstricker, 1931) and will likely be disproportionately affected by COVID-19. Social inequalities such as poverty contribute to conditions that increase the risk of respiratory and other infections (Quinn & Kumar, 2014). For example, urban poverty is associated with poor housing conditions (e.g., household crowding, mold, poor indoor air quality; Blumenshine et al., 2008; Rauh et al., 2008), which increase the risk of various health problems and transmission of respiratory infections (Krieger & Higgins, 2002; Rauh et al., 2008). In addition, the recommended precautionary measures against COVID-19 including frequent hand washing, disinfecting households, or social distancing (Centers for Disease Control and Prevention, 2020b) require access to basic resources, such as housing and water. The World Health Organization reported that "2.0 billion people still do not have basic sanitation facilities such as toilets or latrines" (World Health Organization, 2019, Key facts section) and "827,000 people in low-and middle-income countries die as a result of inadequate water, sanitation, and hygiene each year" (World Health Organization, 2019, Sanitation and health section, para. 1). Therefore, proper personal hygiene is a privilege that not everyone has access to.

In addition, socio-demographic factors such as employment, level of wealth, social status, and population density can affect individuals' ability to adopt social distancing practices. Based on the results of a cell-phone location data analysis, the New York Times reported that wealthy people in the United States were more likely than poor people to stay at home during the workweek and began implementing social distancing practices earlier than poor people (Valentino-DeVries et al., 2020). Several news sources reported that many well-off NYC residents fled to their vacation homes after the rapid spread of COVID-19 in New York City (NYC) in March 2020, but fleeing from NYC was not an option for many NYC residents, including lower-income workers who were unable to risk losing their jobs and had to continue to go to work. Therefore, while wealthier people are not invulnerable to COVID-19, they may have a greater ability to protect themselves from it.

The relationship between social disadvantage and COVID-19 has yet to be fully understood; however, preliminary data published by the New York City Department of Health and Mental Hygiene (2020) indicated that a disproportionately high number of COVID-19 cases were reported in low-income neighborhoods in NYC. In addition, as of April 24, age-adjusted COVID-19 death rates were approximately twice as high among Hispanic/Latinx and Black/African American populations as among White and Asian populations (New York City Department of Health and Mental Hygiene, 2020). Early data from other states such as Illinois, Louisiana, and Michigan also suggest that COVID-

19 has disproportionately affected racial minorities. For example, as of April 26, Blacks/African Americans accounted for more than half of COVID-19 deaths in Chicago (City of Chicago, 2020). According to the preliminary data published by the Centers for Disease Control and Prevention (2020c), non-Hispanic Blacks accounted for approximately one-third of the COVID-19-related hospitalizations as of April 18.

Socially disadvantaged individuals currently experience and will likely continue to experience various additional stressors that may increase the risk of PTSD. While many people have suffered financial losses (e.g., business closures, job loss, reduced work hours) during the past few months, CUNY's weekly survey of NYC residents indicated that Hispanic/Latinx and low-income residents were more likely than other ethnic or racial groups and higher-income residents to lose their jobs (CUNY Graduate School of Public Health and Health Policy, 2020b). As of April 12, housing-related stressors, such as inability to pay rent and fear of being evicted were more common among Hispanic/Latinx and Black/African American residents than among White/European and Asian residents (CUNY Graduate School of Public Health and Health Policy, 2020d). In addition, Hispanic/Latinx residents were more likely than other racial groups to report other stressors, such as social isolation (CUNY Graduate School of Public Health and Health Policy, 2020c) and loss of health insurance (CUNY Graduate School of Public Health and Health Policy, 2020e).

Job loss, loss of health insurance coverage, social isolation, and housing-related stressors can increase the risk of PTSD and chronic psychological distress. For example, experiencing unemployment following the September 11 attacks was a significant predictor of persistent PTSD (Nandi et al., 2004). In addition, studies that examined the psychological consequences of natural disasters reported that low social support, financial losses, and greater exposure to disaster-related stressors (including housing problems) were associated with both increased risk of developing PTSD and more persistent symptoms of PTSD (Galea et al., 2008; Lowe et al., 2015).

Taken together, social inequalities lead to unequal exposure to risk factors. The early data from the United States show that both exposure-related risk factors and pandemic-related stressors are more prevalent among socially disadvantaged populations. The cumulative effects of these risk factors can be devastating and may place disadvantaged populations at high risk for developing PTSD and chronic psychological distress.

Living with a disability

Individuals with disabilities who have limited mobility or have difficulty understanding or communicating information may not only be at high risk of contracting COVID-19 (Centers for Disease Control and Prevention, 2020a), but may also experience unique challenges and stressors during this pandemic. For example, individuals living with severe spinal cord injuries (SCIs) are at heightened risk of respiratory or other infections, as well as the complications from these infections due to reduced immune capacity (Bracchi-Ricard et al., 2016; Brommer et al., 2016; Campagnolo et al., 1994; Held et al., 2010) and impaired respiratory function (Zimmer et al., 2007). In addition, keeping a safe distance from others is difficult for individuals with SCIs and other disabilities who need assistance with self-care and daily activities; thus, these individuals may experience greater fear of being infected. According to news sources, many individuals with severe disabilities also fear that they could be denied treatment (e.g., ventilator support) due to their disability if hospitals are overwhelmed and unable to provide life-saving treatment to all COVID-19 patients. These fears can have profound and long-lasting effects on their mental health.

Individuals with disabilities who need assistance with self-care may experience various additional stressors, such as disruptions in support and services (e.g., if their caregivers are unable to work or become infected; for a discussion, see Campbell et al., 2009) and difficulty accessing vital supplies. After the COVID-19 outbreak began, accessing food and basic supplies have become difficult in many parts of the world due to panic shopping and supermarkets and stores not being able to meet the increased demand. The increased use of online supermarket deliveries has resulted in significant delivery delays, and securing a home-delivery slot has become increasingly difficult. These problems may not only increase the distress of individuals with disabilities who rely on home deliveries but may also affect their physical health and their ability to survive.

Persons with disabilities have been largely overlooked in previous studies that examined the mental health effects of infectious disease outbreaks. Accordingly, there is limited information on their specific needs and psychological experiences. Campbell et al. (2009) reported that individuals with disabilities are disproportionately affected during natural disasters and may also be at high risk during infectious disease pandemics because public health planning and emergency response systems are not prepared to adequately address the needs of this population. Thus, it is important that future studies on COVID-19 focus on specific needs and experiences of individuals with disabilities in order to inform policy and practice.

Occupational group and job responsibilities

Some individuals are at high risk of being exposed to COVID-19 due to their occupation or job responsibilities. While working remotely from home has become the norm during the COVID-19 outbreak, essential business workers, many of whom are low-wage workers, have continued to work on-site; thus, they may not only be at high risk of contracting COVID-19, but may also experience more fears and anxiety (e.g., fear of becoming infected and fear of infecting their loved ones). In addition, first responders and medical workers may be disproportionately affected by COVID-19.

Due to the rapid spread of COVID-19 worldwide, the health-care systems of several countries across the world have been overwhelmed and health-care workers, particularly those who provide direct care to individuals with COVID-19 in overburdened areas, have been experiencing significant physical and psychological strain. A paper published in March 2020 indicated that approximately 20% of the health-care workers who work in hospitals in Lombardy, the most affected region of Italy, have contracted COVID-19 and some of them lost their lives (Remuzzi & Remuzzi, 2020). In addition, news sources reported that two health-care workers who had worked on the front line of the COVID-19 outbreak in Italy committed suicide.

Researchers who have begun to study health-care workers' psychological reactions to the COVID-19 pandemic have reported a high prevalence of distress among front-line health-care workers (Lai et al., 2020). In a recent survey of 1257 nurses and physicians in Wuhan and other cities in China, the vast majority of the participants reported some symptoms of intrusion, avoidance, or hyperarousal (71.5%) and half of them (50.4%) reported depressive symptoms. The prevalence of severe distress (i.e., intrusion, avoidance, and hyperarousal symptoms) was 12.6% among health-care workers in Wuhan and 7.2% among those outside of Wuhan. The results of this study also indicated that working on the front line of the COVID-19 outbreak, being a nurse (vs. being a physician), being a woman, and working in Wuhan (vs. other areas in Hubei province or outside of Hubei province) were associated with higher scores on all indicators of distress (Lai et al., 2020).

Previous studies that examined the mental health consequences of the SARS outbreak reported a heightened risk of PTSD among health-care workers (Lin et al., 2007; Reynolds et al., 2008). A study conducted after the SARS outbreak in Taiwan (Lin et al., 2007) reported that the prevalence of PTSD was 21.7% among doctors and nurses who worked in an emergency department and 13% among those who worked in a psychiatric ward. Health-care workers who experienced quarantine during the SARS outbreak in Canada reported higher levels of posttraumatic stress than the general population who were placed in quarantine (Reynolds et al., 2008). In another study conducted in Hong Kong, health-care worker survivors of SARS reported significantly higher depression, anxiety, stress, and posttraumatic stress one year after the SARS outbreak than SARS survivors who were not health-care workers (Lee et al., 2007).

Gender

Both earlier findings (Hong et al., 2009; Mak et al., 2010) and recent research (Lai et al., 2020; Liu et al., 2020; Sun et al., 2020) suggest that women might be at higher risk of developing PTSD following infectious disease outbreaks than men. The recent COVID-19 literature has highlighted this gender difference in PTSD among health care workers (Lai et al., 2020) and the general adult population (Liu et al., 2020; Sun et al., 2020). In addition, previous research indicated that women survivors of SARS were more likely to develop PTSD and/or chronic psychological dysfunction than men survivors (Bonanno et al., 2008; Hong et al., 2009; Mak et al., 2010). For example, Hong et al. (2009) reported that 26.1% of men and 53.3% of women developed PTSD at some point after being hospitalized for SARS. These findings are consistent with broader trauma literature which suggests that the risk of PTSD is twice as high among women as among men (Tolin & Foa, 2006).

Age

Older adults were more likely to report elevated PTSD symptomatology than middle-aged adults following the SARS outbreak (Lee et al., 2006). In addition, Yip et al. (2010) highlighted the increased suicide rates among older adults (65 years of age and older) following the SARS outbreak in Hong Kong and reported a link between SARS-related suicides and social isolation (or fear of social isolation), fear of becoming infected with SARS, and feelings of being a burden to one's family among older adults. Our knowledge of the psychological impact of COVID-19 on older adults is limited; however, preliminary data from the United States indicate that hospitalization rates from COVID-19 are highest among older adults aged 65 and older (Centers for Disease Control and Prevention, 2020c). Given that hospitalization for COVID-19 might be a risk factor for PTSD and chronic psychological distress, providing support and professional psychological help to older adults who have been quarantined and/or hospitalized for COVID-19 may be of critical importance.

In addition, according to CUNY's weekly survey results, older adults (over 60 years of age) felt more socially isolated than younger adults (18-29 years old) after the COVID-19 outbreak in NYC (CUNY Graduate School of Public Health and Health Policy, 2020a). However, despite feeling more isolated, older adults reported less anxiety, depression, and hopelessness than younger adults (CUNY Graduate School of Public Health and Health Policy, 2020c). Similar to these results, a recent study indicated that older adults experienced less post-traumatic stress than younger adults after the COVID-19 outbreak in China (Jiang et al., 2020). While these findings suggest that the presence of certain risk factors (i.e., older age, social isolation) alone may not automatically lead to poorer mental health outcomes, it is important to examine longer-term psychological effects of COVID-19 and social isolation among older adults. As previously noted, some individuals who initially demonstrate positive adjustment can later develop psychological problems (Bonanno et al., 2008). Bonanno et al. (2008) found that SARS survivors who exhibited delayed psychological reactions had lower social support than those who consistently reported positive psychological functioning. Therefore, social isolation and loneliness can take a toll in the long run.

It is also important to examine how different risk and protective factors may interact in predicting individuals' responses to the COVID-19 pandemic. Although older age is associated with certain risk factors, older adults may be less likely than younger adults to experience certain pandemic-related stressors (e.g., job loss, fear of losing one's job, having to go to work). CUNY's COVID-19 survey indicated that younger NYC residents were more likely than older residents to have someone in their household with COVID-19 symptoms and to perceive their chance of being infected as high (CUNY Graduate School of Public Health and Health Policy, 2020b). In addition, 34% of NYC residents who participated in this survey between April 10 and 12 reported that they were not able to pay their rent or mortgage in April and 62% of these participants reported fears of being evicted; however, these stressors were least common in older residents (CUNY Graduate School of Public Health and Health Policy, 2020d). Therefore, it is important to consider potential risk and protective factors that may affect the relationship between age and psychological outcomes.

Conclusions

While many individuals do not develop PTSD or chronic psychological problems after infectious disease outbreaks, as Horesh and Brown (2020) stated, "when we are faced with mass trauma, such as COVID-19, even a significant minority of traumatized individuals will mean that the mental health burden will be enormous" (p. 333). Therefore, identifying the risk factors for PTSD and chronic psychological distress related to COVID-19 is critical in terms of reducing the mental health burden of COVID-19. Increased knowledge of risk factors can allow early detection and treatment of symptoms of PTSD, which may play a critical role in improving long-term mental health outcomes of high-risk populations.

Although the COVID-19 pandemic is unique in several ways and mental health risks associated with COVID-19 have yet to be understood, our review of early data on COVID-19 and previous literature suggest that socio-demographic factors (e.g., gender, age), exposure-related factors (e.g., living in highly affected areas, knowing or having a close relationship with someone infected with COVID-19, becoming infected with COVID-19, being quarantined or hospitalized for COVID-19, and working on the front line of the COVID-19 pandemic), loss of a loved one, and pandemic-related worries and stressors (e.g., fear of being infected, concerns about family members' health and safety, financial losses, job loss, housing problems, social isolation and lack of support) may contribute to an increased risk of PTSD and chronic psychological distress. In addition, some populations, such as individuals with certain disabilities may experience unique challenges and stressors during the COVID-19 pandemic, which may place them at high risk of developing PTSD and chronic psychological distress.

The initial data from the United States indicate that several of the risk factors we reviewed in this study have disproportionately affected low-income, Hispanic/Latinx, and African American populations. Therefore, increasing these populations' access to timely mental health care and other resources is of critical importance. In addition, although research has consistently shown that socially disadvantaged individuals are disproportionately affected during infectious disease epidemics and pandemics (e.g., infection rates and mortality rates), there is limited information on the psychological impact of these experiences on these individuals. Most of the previous research in this area, as well as recent COVID-19 studies, have focused on the general population of adults, health-care workers, and hospitalized or quarantined individuals and provided valuable insights into potential risk factors for PTSD and chronic psychological distress. However, it is important that future COVID-19 studies also focus on other populations who might be at high risk (e.g., low-income populations, persons of color, individuals with disabilities, essential business workers, individuals who experience homelessness) in order to inform policy and practice.

It is important to note that we primarily focused on SARS literature and recent preliminary data on COVID-19 in this paper. Other risk factors that have been reported in the broader trauma literature, such as pre-trauma factors including preexisting psychiatric conditions and a tendency to engage in rumination and avoidance coping (for a review, see DiGangi et al., 2013) may interact with the aforementioned risk factors, rendering individuals more vulnerable to PTSD and chronic distress. It is also important to re-emphasize that many individuals maintain positive psychological functioning or experience short-term distress following traumatic events despite the presence of certain risk factors (Bonanno, 2004; Bonanno et al., 2008). Therefore, a comprehensive examination of risk and protective factors can provide valuable insights into the variability of individuals' responses to COVID-19.

References

Blumenshine, P., Reingold, A., Egerter, S., Mockenhaupt, R., Braveman, P., & Marks, J. (2008). Pandemic influenza planning in the United States from a health disparities perspective. *Emerging Infectious Diseases*, *14*(5), 709–715. https://doi.org/10.3201/eid1405.071301

Bo, H.-X., Li, W., Yang, Y., Wang, Y., Zhang, Q., Cheung, T., Wu, X., & Xiang, Y.-T. (2020). Posttraumatic stress symptoms and attitude toward crisis mental health services among clinically stable patients with COVID-19 in China. *Psychological Medicine*. Advance online publication. https://doi.org/10.1017/S0033291720000999

Bonanno, G. A. (2004). Loss, trauma, and human resilience: Have we underestimated the human capacity to thrive after extremely aversive events? *American Psychologist*, *59*(1), 20–28. https://doi.org/10.1037/0003-066X.59.1.20

Bonanno, G. A., Ho, S. M. Y., Chan, J. C. K., Kwong, R. S. Y., Cheung, C. K. Y., Wong, C. P. Y., & Wong, V. C. W. (2008). Psychological resilience and dysfunction among hospitalized survivors of the SARS epidemic in Hong Kong: A latent class approach. *Health Psychology*, *27*(5), 659–667. https://doi.org/10.1037/0278-6133.27.5.659

Bracchi-Ricard, V., Zha, J., Smith, A., Lopez-Rodriguez, D. M., Bethea, J. R., & Andreansky, S. (2016). Chronic spinal cord injury attenuates influenza virus-specific antiviral immunity. *Journal of Neuroinflammation*, *13*(1), 125. https://doi.org/10.1186/s12974-016-0574-y

Brommer, B., Engel, O., Kopp, M. A., Watzlawick, R., Müller, S., Prüss, H., Chen, Y., DeVivo, M. J., Finkenstaedt, F. W., Dirnagl, U., Liebscher, T., Meisel, A., & Schwab, J. M. (2016). Spinal cord injury-induced immune deficiency syndrome enhances infection susceptibility dependent on lesion level. *Brain*, *139*(3), 692–707. https://doi.org/10.1093/brain/awv375

Brooks, S. K., Webster, R. K., Smith, L. E., Woodland, L., Wessely, S., Greenberg, N., & Rubin, G. J. (2020). The psychological impact of quarantine and how to reduce it: Rapid review of the evidence. *The Lancet, 395*(10227), 912–920. https://doi.org/10.1016/S0140-6736(20)30460-8

Campagnolo, D. I., Keller, S. E., DeLisa, J. A., Glick, T. J., Sipski, M. L., & Schleifer, S. J. (1994). Alteration of immune system function in tetraplegics. A pilot study. *American Journal of Physical Medicine & Rehabilitation, 73*(6), 387–393. https://doi.org/10.1097/00002060-199411000-00003

Campbell, V. A., Gilyard, J. A., Sinclair, L., Sternberg, T., & Kailes, J. I. (2009). Preparing for and responding to pandemic influenza: Implications for people with disabilities. *American Journal of Public Health, 99*(S2), S294–S300. https://doi.org/10.2105/AJPH.2009.162677

Centers for Disease Control and Prevention. (2017, December 6). *Severe acute respiratory syndrome (SARS): SARS basic fact sheet.* CDC. https://www.cdc.gov/sars/about/fs-sars.html

Centers for Disease Control and Prevention. (2020a, April 7). *Coronavirus disease 2019 (COVID-19): People with disabilities.* CDC. https://www.cdc.gov/coronavirus/2019-ncov/need-extra-precautions/people-with-disabilities.html

Centers for Disease Control and Prevention. (2020b, April 8). *Coronavirus disease 2019 (COVID-19): How to protect yourself & others.* CDC. https://www.cdc.gov/coronavirus/2019-ncov/prevent-getting-sick/prevention.html

Centers for Disease Control and Prevention. (2020c, April 24). *COVIDView: A weekly surveillance summary of U.S. COVID-19 activity.* CDC. https://www.cdc.gov/coronavirus/2019-ncov/covid-data/covidview/index.html

City of Chicago. (2020, April 26). *Latest data.* City of Chicago. https://www.chicago.gov/content/city/en/sites/covid-19/home/latest-data.html

CUNY Graduate School of Public Health and Health Policy. (2020a). *COVID-19 tracking survey.* CUNY. https://sph.cuny.edu/research/covid-19-tracking-survey/

CUNY Graduate School of Public Health and Health Policy. (2020b). *CUNY New York City COVID-19 survey week 3.* CUNY. https://sph.cuny.edu/research/covid-19-tracking-survey/week-3/

CUNY Graduate School of Public Health and Health Policy. (2020c). *CUNY New York City COVID-19 survey week 4.* CUNY. https://sph.cuny.edu/research/covid-19-tracking-survey/week-4/

CUNY Graduate School of Public Health and Health Policy. (2020d). *CUNY New York City COVID-19 survey week 5.* CUNY. https://sph.cuny.edu/research/covid-19-tracking-survey/week-5/

CUNY Graduate School of Public Health and Health Policy. (2020e). *CUNY New York City COVID-19 survey week 7.* CUNY. https://sph.cuny.edu/research/covid-19-tracking-survey/week-7/

DiGangi, J. A., Gomez, D., Mendoza, L., Jason, L. A., Keys, C. B., & Koenen, K. C. (2013). Pretrauma risk factors for posttraumatic stress disorder: A systematic review of the literature. *Clinical Psychology Review, 33*(6), 728–744. https://doi.org/10.1016/j.cpr.2013.05.002

Galea, S., Tracy, M., Norris, F., & Coffey, S. F. (2008). Financial and social circumstances and the incidence and course of PTSD in Mississippi during the first two years after Hurricane Katrina. *Journal of Traumatic Stress, 21*(4), 357–368. https://doi.org/10.1002/jts.20355

Gamino, L. A., Easterling, L. W., Stirman, L. S., & Sewell, K. W. (2000). Grief adjustment as influenced by funeral participation and occurrence of adverse funeral events. *OMEGA - Journal of Death and Dying*, *41*(2), 79–92. https://doi.org/10.2190/QMV2-3NT5-BKD5-6AAV

Gardner, P., & Moallef, P. (2015). Psychological impact on SARS survivors: Critical review of the English language literature. *Canadian Psychology/Psychologie Canadienne*, *56*(1), 123–135. https://doi.org/10.1037/a0037973

Hawryluck, L., Gold, W. L., Robinson, S., Pogorski, S., Galea, S., & Styra, R. (2004). SARS control and psychological effects of quarantine, Toronto. *Emerging Infectious Diseases*, *10*(7), 1206–1212. https://doi.org/10.3201/eid1007.030703

Held, K. S., Steward, O., Blanc, C., & Lane, T. E. (2010). Impaired immune responses following spinal cord injury lead to reduced ability to control viral infection. *Experimental Neurology*, *226*(1), 242–253. https://doi.org/10.1016/j.expneurol.2010.08.036

Hong, X., Currier, G. W., Zhao, X., Jiang, Y., Zhou, W., & Wei, J. (2009). Posttraumatic stress disorder in convalescent severe acute respiratory syndrome patients: A 4-year follow-up study. *General Hospital Psychiatry*, *31*(6), 546–554. https://doi.org/10.1016/j.genhosppsych.2009.06.008

Horesh, D., & Brown, A. D. (2020). Traumatic stress in the age of COVID-19: A call to close critical gaps and adapt to new realities. *Psychological Trauma: Theory, Research, Practice and Policy*, *12*(4), 331–335. https://doi.org/10.1037/tra0000592

Jiang, H., Nan, J., Lv, Z., & Yang, J. (2020). Psychological impacts of the COVID-19 epidemic on Chinese people: Exposure, post-traumatic stress symptom, and emotion regulation. *Asian Pacific Journal of Tropical Medicine*. Advance online publication. http://www.apjtm.org/preprintarticle.asp?id=281614

Keyes, K. M., Pratt, C., Galea, S., McLaughlin, K. A., Koenen, K. C., & Shear, M. K. (2014). The burden of loss: Unexpected death of a loved one and psychiatric disorders across the life course in a national study. *American Journal of Psychiatry*, *171*(8), 864–871. https://doi.org/10.1176/appi.ajp.2014.13081132

Krieger, J., & Higgins, D. L. (2002). Housing and health: Time again for public health action. *American Journal of Public Health*, *92*(5), 758–768. https://doi.org/10.2105/AJPH.92.5.758

Kwek, S.-K., Chew, W.-M., Ong, K.-C., Ng, A. W.-K., Lee, L. S.-U., Kaw, G., & Leow, M. K.-S. (2006). Quality of life and psychological status in survivors of severe acute respiratory syndrome at 3 months postdischarge. *Journal of Psychosomatic Research*, *60*(5), 513–519. https://doi.org/10.1016/j.jpsychores.2005.08.020

Lai, J., Ma, S., Wang, Y., Cai, Z., Hu, J., Wei, N., Wu, J., Du, H., Chen, T., Li, R., Tan, H., Kang, L., Yao, L., Huang, M., Wang, H., Wang, G., Liu, Z., & Hu, S. (2020). Factors associated with mental health outcomes among health care workers exposed to coronavirus disease 2019. *JAMA Network Open*, *3*(3), e203976. https://doi.org/10.1001/jamanetworkopen.2020.3976

Lau, J. T. F., Yang, X., Pang, E., Tsui, H. Y., Wong, E., & Wing, Y. K. (2004). SARS-related perceptions in Hong Kong. *Emerging Infectious Diseases*, *10*(4), 587–424. https://doi.org/10.3201/eid1103.040675 https://doi.org/10.3201/eid1004.030628

Lee, A. M., Wong, J. G. W. S., McAlonan, G. M., Cheung, V., Cheung, C., Sham, P. C., Chu, C.-M., Wong, P.-C., Tsang, K. W. T., & Chua, S. E. (2007). Stress and psychological distress among SARS survivors 1 year after the outbreak. *The Canadian Journal of Psychiatry*, *52*(4), 233–240. https://doi.org/10.1177/070674370705200405

Lee, T. M. C., Chi, I., Chung, L. W. M., & Chou, K.-L. (2006). Ageing and psychological response during the post-SARS period. *Aging & Mental Health, 10*(3), 303–311. https://doi.org/10.1080/13607860600638545

Liao, Q., Cowling, B. J., Lam, W. W. T., Ng, D. M. W., & Fielding, R. (2014). Anxiety, worry and cognitive risk estimate in relation to protective behaviors during the 2009 influenza A/H1N1 pandemic in Hong Kong: Ten cross-sectional surveys. *BMC Infectious Diseases, 14*(1), 169. https://doi.org/10.1186/1471-2334-14-169

Limcaoco, R. S. G., Mateos, E. M., Fernandez, J. M., Roncero, C. (2020). *Anxiety, worry and perceived stress in the world due to the COVID-19 pandemic, March 2020. Preliminary results.* MedRxiv. https://doi.org/10.1101/2020.04.03.20043992

Lin, C.-Y., Peng, Y.-C., Wu, Y.-H., Chang, J., Chan, C.-H., & Yang, D.-Y. (2007). The psychological effect of severe acute respiratory syndrome on emergency department staff. *Emergency Medicine Journal, 24*(1), 12–17. https://doi.org/10.1136/emj.2006.035089

Liu, N., Zhang, F., Wei, C., Jia, Y., Shang, Z., Sun, L., Wu, L., Sun, Z., Zhou, Y., Wang, Y., & Liu, W. (2020). Prevalence and predictors of PTSS during COVID-19 outbreak in China hardest-hit areas: Gender differences matter. *Psychiatry Research, 287*, 112921. https://doi.org/10.1016/j.psychres.2020.112921

Lowe, S. R., Sampson, L., Gruebner, O., & Galea, S. (2015). Psychological resilience after Hurricane Sandy: The influence of individual- and community-level factors on mental health after a large-scale natural disaster. *PLoS One, 10*(5), e0125761. https://doi.org/10.1371/journal.pone.0125761

Mak, I. W. C., Chu, C. M., Pan, P. C., Yiu, M. G. C., Ho, S. C., & Chan, V. L. (2010). Risk factors for chronic post-traumatic stress disorder (PTSD) in SARS survivors. *General Hospital Psychiatry, 32*(6), 590–598. https://doi.org/10.1016/j.genhosppsych.2010.07.007

Mamelund, S.-E., (2004). *An egalitarian disease? Socioeconomic status and individual survival of the Spanish Influenza pandemic of 1918–19 in the Norwegian capital of Kristiania (Memorandum 2004,06).* University of Oslo.

Nandi, A., Galea, S., Tracy, M., Ahern, J., Resnick, H., Gershon, R., & Vlahov, D. (2004). Job loss, unemployment, work stress, job satisfaction, and the persistence of posttraumatic stress disorder one year after the September 11 attacks. *Journal of Occupational and Environmental Medicine, 46*(10), 1057–1064. https://doi.org/10.1097/01.jom.0000141663.22902.0a

New York City Department of Health and Mental Hygiene. (2020, April 24). *COVID-19: Data.* New York City. https://www1.nyc.gov/site/doh/covid/covid-19-data.page

New York State Department of Health. (2020a, April 26). *Fatalities.* NYSDH. https://covid19tracker.health.ny.gov/views/NYS-COVID19-Tracker/NYSDOHCOVID-19Tracker-Fatalities?%3Aembed=yes&%3Atoolbar=no&%3Atabs=n

New York State Department of Health. (2020b, April 26). *New York State Department of Health COVID-19 tracker.* NYSDH. https://covid19tracker.health.ny.gov/views/NYS-COVID19-Tracker/NYSDOHCOVID-19Tracker-Map?%3Aembed=yes&%3Atoolbar=no&%3Atabs=n

Petrosillo, N., Viceconte, G., Ergonul, O., Ippolito, G., & Petersen, E. (2020). COVID-19, SARS and MERS: Are they closely related? *Clinical Microbiology and Infection.* Advance online publication. https://doi.org/10.1016/j.cmi.2020.03.026

Quinn, S. C., & Kumar, S. (2014). Health inequalities and infectious disease epidemics: A challenge for global health security. *Biosecurity and Bioterrorism: Biodefense Strategy, Practice, and Science, 12*(5), 263–273. https://doi.org/10.1089/bsp.2014.0032

Quinn, S. C., Kumar, S., Freimuth, V. S., Musa, D., Casteneda-Angarita, N., & Kidwell, K. (2011). Racial disparities in exposure, susceptibility, and access to health care in the US

H1N1 influenza pandemic. *American Journal of Public Health, 101*(2), 285–293. https://doi.org/10.2105/AJPH.2009.188029

Rauh, V. A., Landrigan, P. J., & Claudio, L. (2008). Housing and health: Intersection of poverty and environmental exposures. *Annals of the New York Academy of Sciences, 1136*(1), 276–288. https://doi.org/10.1196/annals.1425.032

Remuzzi, A., & Remuzzi, G. (2020). COVID-19 and Italy: What next? *The Lancet, 395*(10231), 1225–1228. https://doi.org/10.1016/S0140-6736(20)30627-9

Reynolds, D. L., Garay, J. R., Deamond, S. L., Moran, M. K., Gold, W., & Styra, R. (2008). Understanding, compliance and psychological impact of the SARS quarantine experience. *Epidemiology and Infection, 136*(7), 997–1007. https://doi.org/10.1017/S0950268807009156

Sprang, G., & Silman, M. (2013). Posttraumatic stress disorder in parents and youth after health-related disasters. *Disaster Medicine and Public Health Preparedness, 7*(1), 105–110. https://doi.org/10.1017/dmp.2013.22

Sun, L., Sun, Z., Wu, L., Zhu, Z., Zhang, F., Shang, Z., Jia, Y., Gu, J., Zhou, Y., Wang, Y., Liu, N., & Liu, W. (2020). *Prevalence and risk factors of acute posttraumatic stress symptoms during the COVID-19 outbreak in Wuhan, China*. MedRxiv. https://doi.org/10.1101/2020.03.06.20032425

Sydenstricker, E. (1931). The Incidence of Influenza among persons of different economic status during the epidemic of 1918. *Public Health Reports, 46*(4), 154–170. https://doi.org/10.2307/4579923

Tolin, D. F., & Foa, E. B. (2006). Sex differences in trauma and posttraumatic stress disorder: A quantitative review of 25 years of research. *Psychological Bulletin, 132*(6), 959–992. https://doi.org/10.1037/0033-2909.132.6.959

Valentino-DeVries, J., Lu, D., Dance, G. J. X. (2020, April 3). Location data says it all: Staying at home during coronavirus is a luxury. *The New York Times*. https://www.nytimes.com/interactive/2020/04/03/us/coronavirus-stay-home-rich-poor.html

Wang, C., Pan, R., Wan, X., Tan, Y., Xu, L., Ho, C. S., & Ho, R. C. (2020). Immediate psychological responses and associated factors during the initial stage of the 2019 Coronavirus Disease (COVID-19) epidemic among the general population in China. *International Journal of Environmental Research and Public Health, 17*(5), 1729. https://doi.org/10.3390/ijerph17051729

Weathers, F. W., Litz, B. T., Herman, D., Huska, J., & Keane, T. M. (1993, October 24-27). *The PTSD Checklist (PCL): Reliability, validity, and diagnostic utility* [Paper presentation]. Annual Convention of the International Society for Traumatic Stress Studies, San Antonio, TX, USA.

World Health Organization. (2019, June 14). *Sanitation*. WHO. https://www.who.int/news-room/fact-sheets/detail/sanitation

World Health Organization. (2020a). *Naming the coronavirus disease (COVID-19) and the virus that causes it*. WHO. https://www.who.int/emergencies/diseases/novel-coronavirus-2019/technical-guidance/naming-the-coronavirus-disease-(covid-2019)-and-the-virus-that-causes-it

World Health Organization. (2020b, January 12). *Novel coronavirus – China*. WHO. http://www.who.int/csr/don/12-january-2020-novel-coronavirus-china/en/

World Health Organization. (2020c, March 11). *WHO Director-General's opening remarks at the media briefing on COVID-19—11 March 2020*. WHO. https://www.who.int/dg/speeches/detail/who-director-general-s-opening-remarks-at-the-media-briefing-on-covid-19—11-march-2020

World Health Organization. (2020d, April 28). *Coronavirus disease (COVID-19) pandemic*. WHO. https://www.who.int/emergencies/diseases/novel-coronavirus-2019

World Health Organization. (2020e, April 28). *Coronavirus disease (COVID-2019) situation reports.* WHO. https://www.who.int/emergencies/diseases/novel-coronavirus-2019/situation-reports

Wu, K. K., Chan, S. K., & Ma, T. M. (2005). Posttraumatic stress after SARS. *Emerging Infectious Diseases, 11*(8), 1297–1300. https://doi.org/10.3201/eid1108.041083

Yip, P. S. F., Cheung, Y. T., Chau, P. H., & Law, Y. W. (2010). The impact of epidemic outbreak: The case of severe acute respiratory syndrome (SARS) and suicide among older adults in Hong Kong. *Crisis, 31*(2), 86–92. https://doi.org/10.1027/0227-5910/a000015

Yu, H. Y. R., Ho, S. C., So, K. F. E., & Lo, Y. L. (2005). Short communication: The psychological burden experienced by Hong Kong midlife women during the SARS epidemic. *Stress and Health, 21*(3), 177–184. https://doi.org/10.1002/smi.1051

Zimmer, M. B., Nantwi, K., & Goshgarian, H. G. (2007). Effect of spinal cord injury on the respiratory system: Basic research and current clinical treatment options. *The Journal of Spinal Cord Medicine, 30*(4), 319–330. https://doi.org/10.1080/10790268.2007.11753947

Managing COVID-19 in a Large Urban Research-Intensive University

Cheryl Regehr and Vivek Goel

ABSTRACT

While universities regularly face emergency situations that affect their operations, the global disruption caused by COVID-19 is unprecedented, presenting unique challenges to universities. This article describes the initial stages of crisis response at a large research-intensive university in the center of a diverse international city. Structural, operational, social/psychological, and communication challenges have shifted during five phases we experienced in COVID-19: preplanning, approaching crisis, immediate crisis, prolonged uncertainty, and planning for restart and recovery. Key to managing challenges is clear but flexible incident management structures, and constant interaction and collaboration among groups addressing varying aspects of the operation.

Universities, and those who lead them, regularly encounter challenging events that affect operations and the health and well-being of their members. These events may include: work stoppages through protests and strikes; health epidemics such as SARS or H1N1; natural disasters such as ice storms and floods; acts of mass violence; economic downturns such as the global recession of 2009; and political upheaval in other parts of the world that influence operations. Indeed, universities prepare for events such as these, and develop plans to address the disruption to operations, maintain core functions, and care for members of their community. Nevertheless, the global disruption caused by COVID-19 is unprecedented, affecting all people across the globe over a prolonged period of time, and presenting challenges to a large research university like the University of Toronto, that have not been seen since the last World War when military tents occupied our playing fields (Friedland, 2013), or perhaps the Spanish Flu of 1919 when schools and universities closed en masse (Stern et al., 2009). That is, COVID-19 represented a true crisis, rather than a routine emergency (Howitt et al., 2009; Leonard & Howitt,

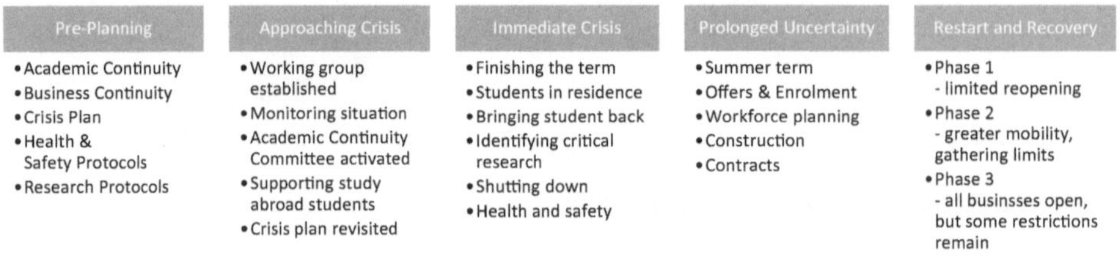

Figure 1. Tasks in COVID-19 crisis management.

2012) requiring novel responses involving all members of the community. Relatively unique in this situation is that the response measures to COVID-19, such as travel restrictions and social distancing measures, are themselves having significant consequences for society that need to be managed, along with the disease itself.

Although what are defined as routine emergencies may be tragic, significantly disrupt operations, and cause harm to individuals, they are within the realm of what is imagined to be possible, and thus standard procedures and responses can be pre-planned. In this way, they are predictable. For instance, horrifying events such as someone with a weapon, injuring or killing others on campus, is one such event for which most institutions of higher learning will have plans (Regehr et al., 2016). Crisis situations similarly affect operations and may cause harm to others, but they are understood to be unpredictable incidents with novel circumstances (Howitt et al., 2009).

Crisis situations, in general, are described to occur in three phases: preplanning and preparation, crisis response, and recovery. The world-wide scale and the ongoing health, political, and economic disruption of COVID-19, however, brought with two additional phases as depicted in Figure 1. One additional phase involved responding to the advancing crisis. A second additional phase was of prolonged uncertainty, during which standard approaches to managing crises were challenged, and during which the impact on members of the community was less predictable than that which occur in a time-limited crisis. While the world has faced major infectious diseases in recent years, such as HIV-AIDS, SARS, MERS, H1N1, and Ebola, this situation is very different. We are faced with a novel, highly contagious virus for which there is no preexisting population immunity, and at present, no proven treatment or vaccine. We have had to resort to global use of public health measures such as travel restrictions and social distancing, as the key pandemic control mechanisms for the first time in a century. Something that is much more challenging given the world is much more interconnected now.

This article describes the initial stages of crisis response in the wake of COVID-19 at a large research-intensive university in the middle of diverse international city. It focuses on some key aspects of the response; other components such as government advocacy, budget analysis and projections, facilities and construction management, and labor relations, are also critical but beyond the scope of this discussion.

The University of Toronto enrolls over 90,000 students across three campuses in the Greater Toronto Area; 22,000 of whom are international students, coming from 163 countries across the world. The University of Toronto is part of a large academic health science collaboration with 12 affiliated partner hospitals. Over $1.4B (Can) of research is conducted per year on campus and in partner hospitals. There are approximately 3000 learners at any given time on placement in health care settings. Fifty-three percent of students are engaged in some sort of experiential learning opportunity. The University also has a broad range of international collaborations with 23% of students studying abroad at some point in their degrees, and over 60 delegations arriving from other institutions each year. In addition, the university hosts a vast number of international events involving academics and political dignitaries, such as the G7 foreign ministers conference.

Pre-planning for crisis and emergency situations

As is the case with other institutions of higher learning, University of Toronto has invested considerable time and energy in developing plans for managing crisis and emergency situations. This pre-planning held us in good stead during the initial periods of the COVID-19 pandemic. In 2018, the University updated its *Policy on Crisis and Routine Emergency Preparedness and Response* which confirmed the University's commitment to "protecting its community, facilities, and property from the effects of routine emergencies and spontaneous, unpredictable crisis situations by establishing specific guidelines, procedures, and resources." Specifically, this policy outlined four priorities for the University in responding to crisis situations: (1) the safety of students, faculty, staff and affected community residents; (2) limiting or containing the extent of damage including making provisions for the safety and protection of research animals and property; (3) ensuring clear and effective communications with members of the community during the situation; (4) recovery and restoration of academic and research operations (University of Toronto Governing Council, 2018).

Supporting the policy is a *Framework for Responding to a Crisis or Routine Emergency* that details responsible individuals, processes, and resources required to respond to challenges. In addition to the overall crisis policy and framework, the University has other aspects of pre-planning that serve in times of crisis including: processes for managing threats of violence (Regehr et al., 2016); a policy on academic continuity (Regehr et al., 2017); business continuity processes; and robust procedures for research integrity and occupational health and safety. These policies, procedures, and processes were developed based on recent experiences, including those of SARS in 2003 in which Toronto was one of the most impacted communities outside of Asia, and the 2009 H1N1 pandemic.

Business continuity

The International Standards Organization defines Business Continuity Management (BCM) as

> a holistic management process that identifies potential impacts that threaten an organisation and provides a framework for building resilience and the capability for an effective response that safeguards the interests of its key stakeholders, reputation, brand and value-creating activities (ISO, 2012)

BCM has been defined as "a process that identifies an organization's exposure to internal and external threats and synthesizes hard and soft assets to provide effective prevention and recovery" (Herbane et al., 2004). BCM involves a process of: risk identification including naturally occurring risks, human error risks, and those arising from malicious acts; evaluation of potential financial losses, reputational damages, and possible legal action; risk mitigation strategies including minimizing risk, transferring risk such as through insurance, and creating redundancies; establishing disaster recovery plans; and developing a process of continuous monitoring and controls (Gibb & Buchanan, 2006). It has alternatively been described as occurring in four phases, protection, mitigation, emergency, and recovery (Zeng & Zio, 2017). BCM has its origins in information technology and only recently has been expanded to include not only the technological but also the social aspects of ensuring the safety of assets and the continuity of operations (Elliott et al., 2010). In the higher education sector, it has also been expanded to consider not only information systems, but also communication channels and program offerings, which can be strengthened through inter-institutional partnerships (Mann, 2007).

Academic continuity

Despite the centrality of academic programs to the mission and financial stability of institutions of higher education, academic continuity has received far less attention than BCM. Nevertheless, institutions have long worked to ensure the continuity of their academic programs during exceptional times. For instance, in 1939 the French government established the *Center national d'enseignement a distance,* and within three months developed correspondence courses in response to disruptions caused by evacuations in WWII (SchWeber, 2008, 2013). More recent examples include Xavier University using Sloan Semester online courses following Hurricane Katrina, the creation of a "virtual residency" involving multimedia approaches by Empire State College in response to the 2006 war in Lebanon (SchWeber, 2013), and the use of online assessment by Canterbury University to replace invigilated assessment following earthquakes in New Zealand (Agnew & Hickson, 2012).

As previously reported (Regehr et al., 2017), the University of Toronto established a *Policy on Academic Continuity* in 2012. The policy clearly outlines the responsibilities of the University for coordinating activity and providing information; academic administrators for overseeing changes and assuming responsibility for courses where an instructor is unavailable; instructors for preparing syllabi in a manner that supports continuity, revising course procedures and requirements, and making reasonable accommodations for students who are unable to attend classes or complete academic requirements; and students for keeping informed and completing all academic requirements. The policy is supported by a process that has been successfully implemented in two previous situations, a labor disruption and the H1N1 pandemic. The first element of the process is pre-planning which involves designing courses for resilience and developing technological systems for online learning and communication. Next, when a crisis is approaching, the continuity committee is activated, information about courses and students at risk is collected, and information about policies and best practices is communicated. During the crisis courses are modified as required, information is shared with faculty and students, and commitment to academic continuity is reiterated. Finally, in the post-crisis period, strategies are reviewed, successes and efforts are acknowledged, and courses continue to be designed for resiliency (Regehr et al., 2017).

Research and health and safety

The *Research Administration Policy* as well as policies and regulatory frameworks on research ethics, animal welfare, biosafety, and occupational health and safety guide the conduct of research. The *Research Oversight and Compliance Office* and *Occupational/Environmental Health and Safety* ensure that all applicable policy and regulatory requirements are met in the workplace, including laboratory settings. These offices also respond to routine emergencies such as power failures, fires, and accidents. Each laboratory is required to have plans in place for disruption of research activities.

The approaching crisis

As the first reports came from China about this new disease, the University of Toronto stepped up its preparatory actions. A working group was established that included representation from student services, occupational health and safety, the study abroad office, the registrar, residence life, and operations, as well as public health expertise. In addition, the Academic Continuity Committee was activated and began meeting on a regular basis. These working groups monitored the situation, developed communications for the community, and supported our students who were in affected regions of the world. They also launched preparations regarding what the university would need to do if there was community transmission of the disease in Canada. These preparations included revisiting the Crisis Policy and Crisis Framework to determine who would need to be engaged if we reached a crisis phase.

On January 25 2020, an individual who had recently returned from Wuhan, China, the epicenter of the COVID-19 pandemic, identified that he was suffering from symptoms of the disease and was placed in isolation in Sunnybrook Hospital, a teaching hospital partner of the University of Toronto. Two days later he was confirmed as Canada's first documented case of coronavirus. Hospital and public health officials acted quickly and unlike during SARS, there was no spread of disease from the early cases, beyond immediate family members. But it was clear that like our experience with SARS, the global links and the volume of international travel, made Canada, and in particular Toronto, vulnerable to an outbreak of coronavirus.

The immediate crisis

During the early days of March, it became increasingly clear that COVID-19 was likely to have a significant effect on university operations and the lives of members of our community. Using a slight modification of the process outlined in our crisis plan, we established a command structure. The authors of this article (Regehr and Goel) served as incident leaders (IL) reporting to the President. Six working groups were established to address academic continuity, student, research, human resources, business continuity, and communications. Leaders of each of the working groups, other vice-presidents, associate vice-presidents and vice-provosts, served on the incident leadership team (ILT), which met daily in the initial stages. The work that had been done over the previous 8 weeks informed the creation of these working groups and enabled them to launch rapidly.

On Wednesday March 11, a notice was sent out to the leaders of all academic divisions reminding them about our commitment to academic and business continuity, and informing them that while Public Health had assessed the risk to the public to be low, we needed to be prepared to enact those plans. Two days later it was announced that the University was taking the unprecedented step of moving all in-person courses to alternative format effective Monday. Residences, libraries, and research operations continued. Despite the view that this was a unique situation, it turned out that this was not unprecedented. Indeed, the "second wave" of the Spanish Flu epidemic hit Toronto in the fall of 1918, causing the University to cancel lectures from October 18 to November 5 (Brown, 2013). As a result, the Senate Committee on the University Library "resolved to close the Reading Room from Oct. 18 to Nov. 4 inclusive, but to keep the building open from 10 a.m. to noon daily for giving out books to students. The south door into the Professors' reading-room remaining open as used during library office-hours." Oddly over 100 years later, we came to a similar conclusion about the University libraries when the City of Toronto ordered all of its libraries to close.

The days following March 11, when the World Health Organization declared a formal pandemic, were complicated by the fact that public health information and government directives shifted on a daily, and sometimes hourly basis. The first indication was a statement from the Provincial Government in the morning of March 12, that families should continue with plans for travel during the public school Spring Break that was set to begin in 2 days. A few hours later, the same government announced that all public schools, from kindergarten to high school, would be closed for 2 weeks following Spring Break. People boarded planes and headed off on holiday. The next day, the City of Toronto closed services including recreational facilities, daycares, and parks, and the Province announced that only businesses on a list of essential services could remain open. On March 14, the Federal Government told Canadians abroad to "get home while they can;" and on March 16, at the tail end of a press conference, Prime Minister Trudeau stated that "Canadians should stay home." The next day, the Premier of Ontario declared a state of emergency.

At that point, we issued a message to all members of our community identifying our commitment to the health and safety of members of our community, but equally our commitment to three core activities during COVID-19: (1) ensuring that our students could complete their terms; (2) providing a safe and welcoming place to live for those students in residence who were unable to return home; and (3) supporting the critical COVID-19 and time-sensitive research endeavors of our world-class researchers. These three priorities formed the basis of our actions and activities in the ensuing weeks.

The University moved students who could return home out of residences, and ensured that the over 3000 who remained, were safe and supported; brought hundreds of study abroad students back from overseas; moved our health and wellness services online; and established emergency bursaries for those student in need. An online absence declaration was implemented in lieu of doctor's note for all students; a process that had proved effective during H1N1 (Regehr et al., 2010). Almost 6400 courses were moved online over one weekend; exams were switched to e-proctoring format or replaced with alternative forms of evaluation; and students were provided with options of credit/no credit in lieu of grades. A process was designed and implemented to identify critical research operations; and those not critical began the arduous process of shutting down. Staff who could, were immediately moved to working from home; critical staff who needed to continue to work at the university were identified and issued formal notices by human resources; and those whose operations were shut down and could not work from home were offered pay continuity. Health and safety personnel responded to all concerns of infection; cleaning and sanitization protocols were ramped up; and critical supplies of personal protective equipment were gathered and shared with our partner hospitals.

People moved quickly into action, demonstrating great creativity, and supporting one another. Faculty members and librarians developed spontaneous mutual aid groups, sharing teaching resources and strategies, and providing grassroots seminars for one another. Students expressed gratitude for the efforts made by staff and faculty through social media and group letters. Resources for supporting research activities from home were identified, such as online information repositories and tools for collaboration. As in the case of SARS in 2003, thousands of health care workers and our health professions post-graduate trainees in our affiliated teaching hospitals "rose to the occasion" and prepared to care for the ill and contain the epidemic (Naylor et al., 2004). Health professional students that were not allowed to continue with their placements in health settings found innovative ways to support the pandemic response as volunteer contact tracers for public health, or providing child care and other supports to health care workers on the frontlines.

At the same time, we were managing fear. At a Campus Council meeting, a student council member sought verification of a report on social media that a fellow student had been removed from campus by people in hazmat suits. There were no cases on campus and certainly no removals of individuals. Some described our student residences as stationary cruise ships (referring to the quarantine of the Diamond Princess off the coast of Japan) (Princess, 2020), urging us to empty residences immediately. These individuals were not taking into account the fact that many students were unable to return to their homes abroad due to travel restrictions and would have been at far greater risk if sent to overcrowd the nearby apartments of friends. They were also unaware or skeptical of the evolving plans to ensure social distancing, modify food service delivery, and facilitate self-isolation in our residences. Some students working in research labs expressed great fear of coming to the university, others that lived in shared off-campus accommodations noted that they felt safer coming to campus than staying at home. Some individuals expressed anger toward, or at times sought to exclude, students and faculty from certain areas of the world, fearing that they may be at higher risk of transmitting illness. This is a phenomenon that has been observed in previous pandemic outbreaks (McCauley et al., 2013).

To some degree health anxiety can be positive and can lead to health-promoting behaviors. Indeed, we used this to good effect earlier in the year when flu vaccine stations were opened across our campuses and student, staff, and faculty alike lined up for vaccines (an interesting phenomenon in itself since they were freely and readily available in most pharmacies that surrounded the campuses). In the case of pandemic, psychological factors are critical to public health strategies of social distancing, hygiene, and vaccination. On the other hand, individuals with high health anxiety can misinterpret benign symptoms as evidence of a serious or fatal illness, leading to an overwhelming of the health system, or maladaptive behaviors (Asmundson & Taylor, 2020). Early data on anxiety related to COVID-19 arose from China, the epicenter of the illness, and demonstrated elevated levels of anxiety in medical staff (Huang et al., 2020), university students (Cao et al., 2020), and the general population (Qiu et al., 2020). For instance, a nation-wide survey in China, which received over 52,000 responses, found moderate to high levels of peritraumatic stress in 35% of respondents, with higher rates among females, those aged 18–30, and those over the age of 60 (Qiu et al., 2020). In Toronto, those individuals in the emergency services and our hospital system, recalled vividly the deaths of health care workers during the SARS pandemic (Loeb et al., 2004).

The communications tasks and challenges were considerable. We worked hard to balance the need for frequent communications to ensure that all members of our community were informed, with the risk of overwhelming people with a large number of communications from various university sources. We implemented a system of consolidated communications vetted through the incident managers to ensure timeliness, streamlining, and consistency of administrative information. But the fear generated by political announcements and media sensationalism was more difficult to combat. To that end, one of the authors (Goel) drew upon his expertise in public health and launched a podcast series on the spread of the pandemic that gained tens of thousands of followers.

Prolonged uncertainty

Unlike many crisis situations such as floods or mass casualties, COVID-19 did not present with an acute emergency situation that ended relatively quickly, allowing the university to move into restart and recovery. Rather, as all readers across the world will know, at the time of this writing, we remain in a global situation of social restrictions, business closures, and closures of public services such as schools, with no indication of when this might end. Thus, both the nature of tasks to be accomplished and the emotional toll on individuals took on a new complexion.

Academic planning focused on preparing a fully online summer term. Unlike the quick move at the end of the winter term, these courses needed to incorporate more sophisticated forms of technology-enhanced learning, requiring investments in technology and significant teaching supports. Students unable to obtain summer jobs and international students who were barred from returning home began registering for the summer term in record numbers, and calls were put out by the large undergraduate divisions for teaching resources from the smaller professional faculties. Information technology personnel ensured that systems could manage the exponential increase in demand from students, staff, and faculty who were remoting into the university. A rich array of online supports for students was developed including accessibility services, health services, study groups, exercise classes, and social clubs. New or revised online summer job opportunities were funded by the university including work-integrated learning (such as developing online course materials), research assistantships, and the creation of a special fund to support creative ideas related to COVID-19 from students. Student bursaries were augmented; student life programs had virtual attendances that surpassed that of all previous face-to-face offerings.

A special $9 M research competition was held over a 4-week period, and 34 projects related to the COVID-19 response were selected for support. University facilities were reconfigured to manufacture critical supplies, evaluate disinfection methods for personal protective equipment, and develop and evaluate technologies such as ventilators and rapid diagnostics. Yet, there were many whose research was derailed, causing anxiety in graduate students, and junior faculty members in particular. From a faculty relations perspective, agreements were made to adjust timelines or processes related to tenure and promotion, student evaluations of courses, and annual merit evaluations. The *School of Graduate Studies* developed guidelines for supervision during COVID-19 and suggestions for alternative research assignments. At the same time, many normal operations, some of which had been put in abeyance, continued or resumed, albeit in more challenging circumstances. These included governance meetings, fall course assignments, budget planning, and admitting students for the fall.

By 4 weeks into the COVID-19 crisis, it became clear that we were moving out of crisis phase in which heightened emotional and physiological response can be adaptive (Caplan, 1964), and into a period of chronic stress in which these same responses become potentially damaging (McEwen & Stellar, 1993; Selye, 1936). One segment of employees was experiencing the strain of increased workload, virtual meetings that relentlessly followed one after the other, and work days that extended well beyond normal hours and were undifferentiated from personal and family time. Another segment of employees was unable to work at all. They feared for their futures, as their operations (such as athletic facilities, catering, and building management) had been fully or mostly shutdown.

Concurrently, life responsibilities continued without regular supports. Parents attempted to home school and entertain their children, while also completing their own assigned work tasks; people with elderly parents dropped groceries at the door, worried for their safety in long-term care facilities, and struggled to maintain homecare services; and family members died without the social and religious rituals to celebrate their lives and comfort the bereaved. For those with strained household relationships, conflicts increased in intensity; those who lived alone were acutely aware of their isolation.

A rapid review published in the Lancet, described the negative psychological effects of pandemics which included post-traumatic stress symptoms, confusion, and anger. These were compounded by the effects of quarantine which included additional problems related to infection fears, frustration, anger, boredom, frustration with inadequate information, financial loss, and stigma (Brooks et al., 2020). A poll commissioned by the Canadian Center on Substance Use and Addiction found that schedule disruptions, boredom, and stress, resulted in increased alcohol consumption in almost a quarter of those between the ages of 18 and 54 (Canadian Center on Substance Use and Addiction, 2020). Other reviews pointed to longer-term outcomes of quarantine including a range of avoidance behaviors with respect to social contact, avoiding closed or public spaces, fear of returning to work, and excessive concerns with hygiene and handwashing (Usher et al., 2020). Trauma researchers warned of the mental health challenges ahead (Pfefferbaum & North, 2020). However, the first research out of China suggested that the imposition of quarantine in and of itself is the not best predictor of negative mental health, rather dissatisfaction with control measures was a critical differentiator (Zhu et al., 2020). Earlier research had similarly found that distress and compliance with quarantine among health care providers in Toronto during the SARS epidemic, was associated with fears of loss of income, logistical challenges such as acquiring groceries, boredom, and a perception that control measures were being inconsistently applied across jurisdictions (DiGiovanni et al., 2004).

While information changed rapidly during the crisis phase, communications and actions followed the ever-changing public health guidelines and were for the most part definitive and directive. During the prolonged uncertainty phase, people looked for answers and direction—when will the campus reopen? will we be able to offer summer camps? what size in-person classes can be offered in the fall? All questions for which no answers existed. We thus re-focused our communications on planning for restart and recovery.

Planning for restart and recovery

As we write this article, the University is in the midst of planning for restart and recovery of operations and the significant adaptation of many different work processes. The Provincial Government has released health and safety guidelines for different work settings. While most employers may only need to consider one or two categories of activity, a university has many more: residences, food services, student services, health centers, trades, libraries, athletics, laboratories, animal care facilities, field stations, and office environments. Travel restrictions affect both teaching and research activities and new approaches to work must be developed.

Factors to be considered in planning for restart span epidemiology, health care capacity, and public health capacity and directives. From an epidemiological perspective, we were watching for decreasing numbers of COVID-19 cases and death. The health care system required sufficient diagnostic testing capacity to manage larger numbers of suspected cases if people were no longer self-isolating, and the ability to manage surge capacity if the number of cases rebounded. Public health measures required the capacity for rapid contact tracing, the ability to quarantine those who cannot be isolated, workplaces and public settings that can accommodate social distancing, and a population willing to follow changing recommendations. In order to safely return to operations at the university, protocols for screening students, employees and visitors, procedures for physical distancing, and policies around use of personal protective equipment would need to be developed, and all members of the community required education on infection control and personal safety.

The restart and recovery planning at University of Toronto has three core elements: (1) repurposing the working groups; (2) creating venues for working across groups to avoid duplication of efforts or working at cross purposes; and (3) providing enhanced information to leaders at all levels across the institution. Recovery and restart from COVID-19 will not happen in one step, but is likely to be uneven, with gradual return to operations, and some setbacks. As a result, plans are focused on a phased return.

At all stages of the COVID-19 crisis, but in particular in planning restart and recovery, activities have required an unprecedented degree of collaboration between parts of the university that traditionally work in silos such as academic divisions, residences, and central services such as student services, human resources, facilities and services, occupational health and safety and campus police. Units such as communications and government relations were required to collaborate with all of these services to keep abreast of a constantly changing environment. Thus, a series of newly designed virtual retreats have been implemented for principal and deans, vice-presidents, and for members of working groups, which are proving to be extremely useful in facilitating collaboration.

In order to enhance communications, a series of slides and presentations in which the university's crisis management structure, the tasks completed, and the current considerations and the tasks underway are being broadly shared, for instance in meetings with hundreds of department chairs, with Chief Administrative Officers across the university, and with residence deans of students. These are serving to assist with a shared understanding, and a degree of comfort that a vast array of considerations about being taken into account. Communications with students focus on preparedness and flexible plans focused on ensuring that they will receive a world-class experience in a safe environment, the character of which will be adapted to new realities. Our communications with government reflect that we are ready for the borders to be reopened, with residence plans, course delivery plans, and health and safety plans to facilitate the safety not only of members of the university, but others in society.

Reflections mid-COVID-19

At this point in this event, we offer a few reflections. As Eisenhower said "plans are worthless, but planning is everything" (Eisenhower, 1957). Our plans helped us to be prepared, but we quickly learned that the typical incident response structure was not appropriate for this type of event. In the early days, we adapted the model, sometimes several times a week. As we have gone through different phases of the event, we have continued to add or remove working groups as well as bringing in different expertise as needed. The typical Incident Management Structure compartmentalizes teams. We have found that we need the opposite—regular opportunities for engagement across teams.

Another new challenge not previously faced has been managing our response remotely. Crisis response teams typically work in command centers that allow for regular interactions and quick convening of different individuals to address pressing issues. Before the move to work from home we worked in this manner, transforming this overnight-required significant adaptation. Team members quickly adapted to using online secure collaboration tools for sharing documents and conducting meetings. However, managing workloads for the teams has been difficult. Each team member is expected to have a back-up that can step in and provide relief. But in a constantly evolving and prolonged situation where almost everyone is working from home it can become difficult to step away and take time off. As we enter our third month, with likely many more to go, this will be a challenge we need to address for our own teams.

As the immediate crisis resolves and we, like the rest of the world, are caught in a prolonged period of uncertainty, coordination in a large, decentralized organization becomes more complex. Leaders across the institution are subject to local pressures and local situational contexts; there is increased pressure for them to act. Establishing overarching plans that consider the various phases and scenarios, and take into account operational details such as the need for and availability of personal protective equipment, the capacity of spaces when social distancing is enforced, and the ability to quarantine students and new faculty arriving from abroad, takes time. Thus, it becomes difficult at times to balance a unified message and set of procedures with local needs. This continues to take extraordinary time and effort.

In summary, COVID-19 is a true crisis situation with novel and ever-changing circumstances that affect all aspects of university operations. We have found that our preexisting policies and protocols have served us well. However, we have managed this far with a structure that is both clear and flexible, with established priorities, and with the good will and hard work of thousands of people dedicated to ensuring the integrity of our academic programs, the care and safety of our students, and to advancing research that will change the course of COVID-19's impact on the world.

ORCID

Vivek Goel http://orcid.org/0000-0002-1389-2007

References

Agnew, S., & Hickson, S. (2012). Using online assessment to replace invigilated assessment in times of natural disaster: Are some online conditions better than others? *Journal of Open, Flexible and Distance Learning, 16*(1), 1–13.

Asmundson, G. J., & Taylor, S. (2020). How health anxiety influences responses to viral outbreaks like COVID-19: What all decision-makers, health authorities, and health care professionals need to know. *Journal of Anxiety Disorders, 71*, 102211. https://doi.org/10.1016/j.janxdis.2020.102211.

Canadian Center on Substance Use and Addiction. (2020). *COVID-19 and increased alcohol consumption: NANOS poll summary report*. COVID-19 and increased alcohol consumption: NANOS Poll Summary Report.

Brooks, S. K., Webster, R. K., Smith, L. E., Woodland, L., Wessely, S., Greenberg, N., & Rubin, G. J. (2020). The psychological impact of quarantine and how to reduce it: Rapid review of the evidence. *The Lancet, 395*(10227), 912–920. https://doi.org/10.1016/S0140-6736(20)30460-8.

Brown, R. (2013). *Arts and science at Toronto: A history, 1827–1990*. University of Toronto Press.

Cao, W., Fang, Z., Hou, G., Han, M., Xu, X., Dong, J., & Zheng, J. (2020). The psychological impact of the COVID-19 epidemic on college students in China. *Psychiatry Research, 287*, 112934. https://doi.org/10.1016/j.psychres.2020.112934.

Caplan, G. (1964). *Principles of preventative psychiatry*. Basic Books.

DiGiovanni, C., Conley, J., Chiu, D., & Zaborski, J. (2004). Factors influencing compliance with quarantine in Toronto during the 2003 SARS outbreak. *Biosecurity and Bioterrorism: Biodefense Strategy, Practice, and Science, 2*(4), 265–272. https://doi.org/10.1089/bsp.2004.2.265.

Eisenhower, D. D. (1957). *Remarks at the National Defense Executive Reserve Conference* [Press release]. https://www.presidency.ucsb.edu/documents/remarks-the-national-defense-executive-reserve-conference

Elliott, D., Swartz, E., & Herbane, B. (2010). *Business continuity management: A crisis management approach*. Routledge.

Friedland, M. L. (2013). *The University of Toronto: A history*. University of Toronto Press.

Gibb, F., & Buchanan, S. (2006). A framework for business continuity management. *International Journal of Information Management, 26*(2), 128–141. https://doi.org/10.1016/j.ijinfomgt.2005.11.008.

Herbane, B., Elliott, D., & Swartz, E. (2004). Business continuity management: Time for a strategic role? *Long Range Planning, 37*(5), 435–457. https://doi.org/10.1016/j.lrp.2004.07.010.

Howitt, A. M., Leonard, H. B., & Giles, D. (2009). *Managing crises*. SAGE.

Huang, J., Han, M., Luo, T., Ren, A., & Zhou, X. (2020). Mental health survey of 230 medical staff in a tertiary infectious disease hospital for COVID-19. *Zhonghua Lao Dong Wei Sheng Zhi ye Bing za Zhi Zhonghua Laodong Weisheng Zhiyebing Zazhi [Chinese Journal of Industrial Hygiene and Occupational Diseases]*, *38*, E001–E001.

ISO. (2012). *Societal security – business continuity management systems – requirements*. http://www.iso.org/iso/news.htm?refid=Ref1587

Leonard, H., & Howitt, A. (2012). Leading in crisis: Observations on the political and decision-making dimensions response. In I. Helsloot, B. Jacobs, & A. Boin (Eds.), *Mega-crises. understanding the prospects, nature, characteristics and the effects of the cataclysmic events* (pp. 25–34). Charles C Thomas Publisher Ltd.

Loeb, M., McGeer, A., Henry, B., Ofner, M., Rose, D., Hlywka, T., Levie, J., McQueen, J., Smith, S., Moss, L., Smith, A., Green, K., & Walter, S. D. (2004). SARS among critical care nurses, Toronto. *Emerging Infectious Diseases*, *10*(2), 251–255. https://doi.org/10.3201/eid1002.030838.

Mann, T. (2007). Strategic and collaborative crisis management: A partnership approach to large-scale crisis. *Planning for Higher Education*, *36*(1), 54–64.

McCauley, M., Minsky, S., & Viswanath, K. (2013). The H1N1 pandemic: Media frames, stigmatization and coping. *BMC Public Health*, *13*(1), 1116. https://doi.org/10.1186/1471-2458-13-1116.

McEwen, B. S., & Stellar, E. (1993). Stress and the individual: Mechanisms leading to disease. *Archives of Internal Medicine*, *153*(18), 2093–2101. https://doi.org/10.1001/archinte.153.18.2093.

Naylor, C. D., Chantler, C., & Griffiths, S. (2004). Learning from SARS in Hong Kong and Toronto. *JAMA*, *291*(20), 2483–2487. https://doi.org/10.1001/jama.291.20.2483.

Pfefferbaum, B., & North, C. S. (2020). Mental health and the COVID-19 pandemic. *New England Journal of Medicine.*

Princess. (2020). *Diamond princess updates: Guest disembarkation complete + team member quarantine.* https://www.princess.com/news/notices_and_advisories/notices/diamond-princess-update.html.

Qiu, J., Shen, B., Zhao, M., Wang, Z., Xie, B., & Xu, Y. (2020). A nationwide survey of psychological distress among Chinese people in the COVID-19 epidemic: Implications and policy recommendations. *General Psychiatry*, *33*(2), e100213. https://doi.org/10.1136/gpsych-2020-100213.

Regehr, C., Glancy, G., Carter, A., Ramshaw, L. (2016). *Institutional Responsibilities: The partnership between forensic psychiatry and higher education in threat assessment* [Paper presentation]. Canadian Academy of Psychiatry and the Law, Vancouver.

Regehr, C., Nelson, S., & Hildyard, A. (2017). Academic continuity planning in higher education. *Journal of Business Continuity & Emergency Planning*, *11*(1), 73–84.

Regehr, C., Swift, K., Leigh, J., Matus, J., & Delaney, J. (2010). Student declarations of absence in lieu of doctor's notes. *Canadian Journal of Public Health Revue Canadienne de Sante Publique*, *101*(2), 186–187. https://doi.org/10.1007/BF03404369.

SchWeber, C. (2008). Determined to learn: Accessing education despite life-threatening disasters. *Journal of Asynchronous Learning Networks*, *12*(1), 37–43.

SchWeber, C. (2013). Survival lessons: Academic continuity, business continuity, and technology. In P. Van den Bossche (Ed.), *In facilitating learning in the 21st century: Leading through technology, diversity and authenticity* (pp. 151–163). Springer.

Selye, H. (1936). A syndrome produced by diverse nocuous agents. *Nature*, *138*(3479), 32–32. https://doi.org/10.1038/138032a0.

Stern, A. M., Cetron, M. S., & Markel, H. (2009). Closing the schools: Lessons from the 1918–19 U.S. influenza pandemic . *Health Aff (Millwood)))*, *28*(6), w1066–w1078. https://doi.org/10.1377/hlthaff.28.6.w1066

University of Toronto Governing Council. (2018). *Policy on crisis and routine emergency preparedness and response.* https://governingcouncil.utoronto.ca/secretariat/policies/crisis-and-routine-emergency-preparedness-and-response-policy-june-27-2018.

Usher, K., Bhullar, N., & Jackson, D. (2020). Life in the pandemic: Social isolation and mental health. *Journal of Clinical Nursing, 00,* 1–2. https://doi.org/10.1111/jocn.15290.

Zeng, Z., & Zio, E. (2017). An integrated modeling framework for quantitative business continuity assessment. *Process Safety and Environmental Protection, 106,* 76–88. https://doi.org/10.1016/j.psep.2016.12.002.

Zhu, S., Wu, Y., Zhu, C. Y., Hong, W. C., Yu, Z. X., Chen, Z. K., Chen, Z. I., Jiang, D. G., & Wang, Y. G. (2020). The immediate mental health impacts of the COVID-19 pandemic among people with or without quarantine managements. *Brain, Behavior, and Immunity,* https://doi.org/10.1016/j.bbi.2020.04.045

Romantic Love in the Age of COVID-19

Susan S. Hendrick and Clyde Hendrick

To have and to hold, to love and to cherish, in sickness and in health …

Whether you are partnered or available—love in the age of the coronavirus is challenging. For anyone who has had a breakup or who has lost a partner to death, this can be an especially lonely time. Yet love—romantic love in this case, can be a wonderful gift—a gift both for the giver and the receiver. This paper presents research on six love styles. Some of these love styles, when embraced individually or in tandem, may help persons and couples cope with the current isolation required by COVID-19.

However, it is important to note that love does not conquer all! General facets of personality, such as introversion or extroversion, can be accentuated under stressful conditions. For example, the enforced seclusion necessitated during critical COVID periods may not be a huge problem for introverts. In fact, this can be a time of renewal, with reading, gardening, or even taking long walks outdoors providing enough stimulation. For extroverts, however, this period can be one of deprivation of all the things that enrich their lives, such as meeting friends for coffee and conversation, exercising at the gym, offering "live" therapy with "live" clients rather than on-screen sessions. Thus, with the caveat that personality is very complicated, we believe that love in a relationship can be of considerable importance during the current world pandemic.

As scholars, we have spent several decades studying and writing about romantic love. We have focused specifically on the love styles as first articulated by Lee (1973). Lee, a sociologist, did extensive research before developing a typology of six different love styles, three of them "primary love styles" and three of them "secondary love styles." Each secondary style is presumably composed of two of the primaries. We have found that in both theory and practice, it is best to think of these love styles simply as six different love styles that are applicable to romantic love.

We decided to measure the love styles as romantic "attitudes," and did considerable research to develop a questionnaire to assess degree of agreement with the six love styles. We assumed that virtually everyone could agree to a greater or lesser extent with the questions reflecting each love style, and therefore people did not have to pick only one style as self-representative. We first published a long form of our scale called the Love Attitudes Scale (LAS) (Adler et al., 1986) and later a shortened form of the scale named the Love Attitudes Scale–Short Form.

The six love styles are Eros (passionate love), Ludus (game-playing love), Storge (friendship-based love), Pragma (practical love), Mania (possessive, dependent love), and Agape (giving love). Although much of our early work was with university students, we also assessed gay and straight men in two geographic locations (Adler et al., 1986), Anglo and Mexican-American couples (Contreras et al., 1996), and others. We have found that groups differ very little if at all in their love styles. The LAS has been used in many countries and has been translated into several languages. Thus, at some level, romantic love appears to be universal.

Our purpose is to propose ways in which these love styles/love attitudes might function in this incredibly challenging "in-your-face" time of COVID. Our goal is to be helpful. As longtime scholars and marital partners (43 years), we are living this pandemic a day at a time, just as you are.

Describing the love styles

The love styles include Eros, Ludus, Storge, Pragma, Mania, and Agape. Eros love is intense, physical, and involves a deep wish to know all about a potential partner immediately. It can sometimes be truly "love at first sight." Ludus love is very different and involves game-playing, having more than one love partner at the same time, and not letting any one person get too close. Storge love is friendship love, sometimes developing out of a long-term friendship or budding from shared attitudes and values. Pragma love is practical love, which we have described as having a "shopping list of qualities" sought in a partner. Mania love is anxious love, wanting a relationship to work yet doubting a partner's affection, while clinging alternately to hope and despair. Finally, Agape love is "gift" love—simply wishing to give a partner the best of oneself and wanting the wellbeing of the partner.

Your love styles

If you are puzzled or annoyed at this point because you experience more than one of these love styles (with the same partner or different partners), we understand. We have described these love styles as relatively "pure types," however we human lovers are complicated and endorse typically a mix of two or more types of love. That is why we developed the Love Attitudes Scale, which allows a respondent to agree more or less with each of the love styles. For the sake of clarity and brevity, we are not going to conjecture about Ludus or Mania in this brief discussion. A pandemic does not lend itself to Ludic game-playing with several different partners. Social distancing except for one's household puts severe limits on us all. The pandemic also makes anxious love just one more anxiety burden that should be "shelved" for the duration of COVID. If you are in a relationship and are experiencing anxiety and doubt about a partner's sincerity, either accept your partner as faithful or press DELETE on the relationship. Do not tie yourself into emotional knots about him or her. Save your energy for family and friends who are part of your household or with whom you have frequent and positive virtual contact. You will have time to be manic when the pandemic is over!

That leaves four love styles about which we can speculate. If Eros is strong in your relationship, then we hope you are together, because being apart could be very stressful. However, if you can stay in close virtual contact, this could be a time for new lovers to gain the deep knowledge about each other that is desired. Hopefully there is some Storge in your relationship because friendship, dependability, and steadiness are extremely important in an intimate relationship, and these qualities are never more important than in times of deep stress (i.e., a pandemic). Being good friends with shared values can be very comforting when the world feels turbulent. Pragma is often under-valued as a love style. Being pragmatic may mean that you have picked a partner carefully or are perhaps waiting to meet a partner who checks most of the boxes on your love shopping list. If your partner has pragmatic tendencies, then you are in luck. Groceries, cooking or take-out, laundry, even working in the yard may be ways in which your partner provides support. Finally, but foremost under our current conditions, is Agape or gift love. Agapic love is realized when the welfare of the partner is equal to or exceeding the welfare of the self. Care and concern are part of agapic love, and agapic giving can help mitigate the enforced closeness and ambient fear of the current pandemic. All four of these love styles/attitudes/behavioral tendencies can be helpful in the time of COVID.

This era of a global pandemic is unfamiliar and frightening to all who view its gravity in a clear-eyed fashion. Yet this is also a time when love and caring (in this case for a romantic partner) can deepen a relationship profoundly. We humans are far from perfect, but loving is in our nature. These love styles offer one way of viewing romantic, partnered love. If you want to know more about these love styles, reach out to us. We will reach back. Meanwhile, take care and be well.

References

Adler, N. J., Hendrick, S. S., & Hendrick, C. (1986). Male sexual preference and attitudes toward love and sexuality. *Journal of Sex Education and Therapy*, *12*(2), 27–30. https://doi.org/10.1080/01614576.1986.11074876

Contreras, R., Hendrick, S. S., & Hendrick, C. (1996). Perspectives on marital love and satisfaction in Mexican American and Anglo-American couples. *Journal of Counseling & Development*, *74*(4), 408–415. https://doi.org/10.1002/j.1556-6676.1996.tb01887.x

Lee, J. A. (1973). *The colors of love: An exploration of the ways of loving*. New Press.

Reaction to the COVID-19 Pandemic: The Influence of Meaning in Life, Life Satisfaction, and Assumptions on World Orderliness and Positivity

Jerzy Trzebiński, Maciej Cabański, and Jolanta Zuzanna Czarnecka

ABSTRACT

The goal of the research was to measure the impact of the meaning in life, life satisfaction, and the beliefs in orderliness and positivity of the social world on emotional and cognitive reactions to the COVID-19 pandemic. The 317 participants were recruited over four days (April 1st–4th) during the start of the dynamic increase of the pandemic in Poland. The study was performed via open-access forums on the internet. The analyses indicated that stronger basic hope and higher levels of meaning in life and life satisfaction correlate with lower state anxiety and lower COVID-19 stress. Mediation analyses suggested the following interpretation of the interdependencies: basic hope supports meaning in life and life satisfaction and the increase in the latter two factors results in lower anxiety and COVID-19 stress. The results suggest that these three global assumptions and feelings may serve as buffers against anxiety as well as nonproductive thinking and decision making in the face of an unpredictable threat.

The ongoing coronavirus pandemic invokes feelings of fear, uncertainty, and anxiety. People have become concerned about the health and even possible death of themselves and others. They fear unemployment, debts, professional career breakdown, and broader economic crisis. The situation is further worsened by an ambivalent attitude to the government agencies which are often seen as both responsible for incidents of disorganization in responding to the pandemic and the only way to find final solutions. In the extreme scenario, the developing pandemic may result in panic reactions, catastrophic interpretation and prediction of events, irrational actions, and—as a consequence—the increasing probability of psychological dysfunctions.

Possible consequences of the COVID-19 pandemic are rather unpredictable in a short and longer perspective because the pandemic is a chain of dangerous, mostly uncontrolled, and dynamic events. In such situations, our thinking and emotions may be influenced not so much by our experience and knowledge but by more general and stable assumptions on the social world and our own lives. These convictions may influence the understanding of incoming facts and simulations of the future—possible, desired, and undesired. Therefore these often hidden and not verbalized convictions may influence our day to day emotions, thinking, and decisions as well as relations with others. On the other hand, although the stop-and-think mindset is an important factor contributing to the influence of general convictions on coping with the threat, the direct pressure of fearful and changing facts may dominate over reflection in these unusual circumstances.

The goal of our research was to observe if the meaning in life, life satisfaction, and the beliefs in orderliness and positivity of the social world have an influence on emotional and cognitive reactions to the COVID-19 pandemic. The hypotheses are that a higher level of meaning in life, own life satisfaction, and strength of belief in the orderliness and positivity of the social environment will partly alleviate strong anxiety and panic reactions and provide a solid background for more reflective and rational behavior in this difficult situation. We expect that the above influence might be observed even under the direct pressure of fearful news on the COVID-19 pandemic. The first two factors, meaning in life and life satisfaction, relate to own person. It might be expected that higher meaning in life together with life satisfaction may provide a psychological buffer against dangerous disorganization. A growing literature documents that higher reports of meaning in life and life satisfaction are associated with better mental and physical health and well-being as well as different aspects of better cognitive and social functioning (Batthyany & Russo-Netzer, 2014; Diener & Biswas-Diener, 2008; Haidt, 2006; Hicks & Routledge, 2013; Seligman, 2002). The evidence suggests that these two kinds of feelings provide a stable, although the often different, basis for the evaluation of personal possibilities and chances to cope with life challenges.

The third factor, beliefs in orderliness and positivity of the social world, is more general. It may be assumed that—because the pandemic has a global character that encompasses the individual experience and is beyond the control of each person—the assumptions about the social world order and positivity might play an important role in influencing attitude toward this event. The name of the third factor—Basic Hope—is taken from Erik Erikson's conceptualization of the first stage of personality development (Erikson, 1968). The level of orderliness in a home environment, predictability of early relationships with parents, as well as the parents' nurturing of the child's needs, are critical factors in the early development of Basic Hope. These presumptions, based on crucial social experiences (Bowlby & Ainsworth, 1965; Bowlby, 1986; Bretherton, 1992), are relatively stable and unverbalized, although they are expressed metaphorically at the individual and social levels (e.g. in the form of religion and ideology). Later social experiences may modify the level of Basic Hope. Basic Hope differs from hope or optimism, which concerns one's future (Seligman, 1991) or personal competencies to achieve goals (Snyder et al., 1999, 2001). Instead, Basic Hope is the basis for future expectations, but these types of expectations are based primarily on how a person understands the world, rather than an assessment of his or her competencies.

Data shows that stronger Basic Hope has various positive consequences (Trzebiński & Zięba, 2004, 2013; Zięba et al., 2010, 2018). It facilitates positive expectations for the future and engagement in searching for solutions to new problems and challenges as well as enforcing trust in partners in social interactions. Basic Hope relates positively to higher openness to experience, readiness for altruistic behavior, and forgiveness for harm. It also results in less severe posttraumatic consequences and relates positively to indications of post-traumatic growth (e.g. in oncology patients and victims of car accidents), as well as in adaptive reactions in cases of irreversible loss and crucial life changes. Conversely, lower Basic Hope is associated with the intensity of depressive thoughts.

To observe how the strength of the meaning in life, life satisfaction, and positive presumptions about the social world influence the levels of situational anxiety and stress due to the developing COVID-19 pandemic we conducted a four-day online survey in the Polish population at the beginning of the pandemic peak.

Background of the study

The study was performed within four days (01.04–04.04). At this time the COVID-19 pandemic was developing rapidly in Poland. According to daily briefings from the government, different medical sources, and mass-media, the number infected by the virus was ever increasing. There was disturbing news on the developing pandemic in neighboring countries. Sources informed about approaching the spreading of the infection. However, the predictions on numbers and different consequences of the pandemic were unclear and changing. There were strong signals of increasing unemployment in many areas of the economy accompanied by the ambiguity of the government's economic policy, which was publicly criticized by the opposition. Schools, universities, and shopping centers had been closed for three weeks and there was limited access to the streets and public places. A recently conducted survey in Poland reveals that 40% of the population reported that they were likely to be infected within the next three months, 38% declared that the eventual infection might end in death, and 59%

stated that the worst is yet to come. Moreover, a comparable number of people are already experiencing the economic ramifications of COVID-19 by reporting difficulties to pay the bills (45%) or mortgage (48%) (Report on COVID-19 in Poland 12th of April, 2020)

Methods

Participants

Invitation to participate in the study was published on open-access forums on the Internet. The 317 participants were recruited in four days from the April 1st—4th, from Wednesday to Saturday. In the beginning, participants were asked about their sex, age, present place of residence, and education.

Procedures

Participants were presented with an explanation of the study: "We invite you to participate in a short, easy, and interesting study. The study addresses the emotions and thoughts evoked by the ongoing coronavirus pandemic, as well as some more general beliefs. We are researchers from the SWPS University in Warsaw. The test takes about 10–15 minutes and consists of completing five short questionnaires. It is on the border of social psychology and sociology. Everyone who participates, if he wants, will receive from us a report with the results and conclusions of the study. The survey is online and is fully anonymous. You can take part at any time. The test does not test knowledge and skills, it only concerns our views and feelings. It's easy to do: you choose one answer—you just choose one answer from several given, the one that best suits your thoughts and feelings. Please choose deliberately and honestly."

Next, participants were presented with five scales: the State-Trait Anxiety Inventory (STAI; Spielberger, 1983), the Satisfaction with Life Scale (SWLS; Diener et al., 1985), the Meaning in Life Scale (MIL), the Basic Hope Scale (BH) and the COVID-19 Stress Scale. The STAI—State scale was always presented first to measure the level of anxiety at that moment, consistently across participants. The next scales were presented in random order. Additionally, the order of the items in the Pandemic Stress scale was randomly assigned.

The Meaning in Life Scale (MIL) includes 8 items selected from the Meaning in Life Questionnaire MLQ—the presence of meaning items (Steger et al., 2006), and the Orientation to Life Questionnaire (Antonovsky, 1987). The instruction is: "Read each of the following statements carefully. Assess how well each of them fits your beliefs and experiences on a 5-point scale where 1 is definitely NOT fitting, 2 – it doesn't really match, 3 – I don't agree or disagree, 4 – it rather matches, 5 – definitely matches."

The scale comprises the following items: *My life makes sense; I have my goals in life and I am attached to them; I am not afraid of my future; There is an order in my life; My past, present and near future combine in a meaningful whole; I would not want to change my current life to another; My views, desires, and decisions are meaningfully interrelated; My life has a clear purpose and deeper meaning*

The Basic Hope Scale (BH) contains 12 statements. The scale has been used in many studies, mostly in the Polish population (Trzebiński & Zięba, 2004 2013; Zięba et al., 2010, 2018). The responses were collected on a 5 point scale where 1 means disagree definitely and 5 means strongly agree.

The scale includes 7 items referring to the world's orderliness: *The world is just and the sooner or later everyone will get what someone deserves; All that happens in the world is or would be explainable; The world is governed by general regularities, although it is sometimes difficult to see and understand them; The world is meaningful and all things have some sense even if we feel lost sometimes; There is some unshakable world order that even the greatest catastrophes and changes cannot threaten; Righteous and good people will be rewarded in some way; Looking from a deeper perspective, even the most incomprehensible railways of human life are explainable and have some sense;* and 5 items referring to the world's positivity: *There will always be some people who will help us in a misfortune; Evil, which is so much around but ultimately will not triumph over good; People can be trusted; The world is good even if we are not doing well; People are good by nature.*

The COVID-19 Stress Scale was constructed by us and contains 16 statements on thoughts and feeling as reactions to the developing COVID-19 pandemic. We were inspired by free experience descriptions by ordinary people in blogs and the internet, as well as reported in mass media a few weeks before the study.

The instruction was: "This questionnaire is about your emotions and thoughts related to the ongoing epidemic and its consequences. The honesty of your answers is important to us. Rate to what extent the following feelings and thoughts caused by the epidemic fits you using a five-point scale from 1 (doesn't fit at all) to 5 (definitely fits)."

Items (order rotated)*: I am more and more afraid for my life and health; I am seriously worried about my professional future; The topic of coronavirus all the time occupies my thoughts; I am overcome with growing terror; I am worried that the long-term consequences of the epidemic will be much worse than we think; I don't know what awaits me and my family in the close future; It seems to me that we will not free ourselves from the epidemic and its effects for several more years; I'm trying to get away from the epidemic*

Table 1. Means, standard deviations, Cronbach's alpha and correlations (Pearson's *r*) of the measured variables *(N = 306)*.

	M	SD	α	1.	2.	3.	4.	5.	6.	7.	8.
1. Gender	...	...		...							
2. Age	31.67	10.74		−0.09	...						
3. BH -orderliness	3.36	0.76	0.75	−0.02	0.08	...					
4. BH - positivity	3.42	0.72	0.69	−0.02	0.19**	0.64***	...				
5. BH - total	3.39	0.67	0.82	−0.03	0.14*	0.94***	0.86***	...			
6. MIL	27.99	6.52	0.87	−0.06	0.21***	0.47***	0.44***	0.50***	...		
7. SWLS	21.63	6.28	0.87	0.00	0.13*	0.36***	0.35***	0.40***	0.75***	...	
8. STAI	57.00	16.63	0.94	0.13*	0.06	−0.14*	−0.14*	−0.16**	−0.26***	−0.27***	...
9. COVID-19 stress	3.05	0.76	0.88	0.14*	0.08	−0.15**	−0.10	−0.14*	−0.28***	−0.21***	0.58***

Notes: Gender coding: 0: Male, 1: Female; BH: Basic Hope; MIL: Meaning in Life; SWLS: Satisfaction with Life Scale; STAI: Anxiety; *$p < .05$; **$p < .01$; ***$p < .001$.

because it makes me panic too much; I am afraid that we will be afraid of contacting each other for a long time; I am afraid that the epidemic will cause the economy to collapse; I have no idea how our country can deal with the consequences of the epidemic; I'm worried that there will be riots in the streets in my country; I am thinking about death more often; I feel an increasing feeling of chaos and hopelessness; I'm afraid that contacts between people will change forever (Control item): *I think that this epidemic is currently the most important problem in our country and Worldwide.*

In the end, we thanked the participants and informed them about the possibility of getting the research report.

Results

Out of 317 participants, eleven participants who strongly disagreed with the statement that the coronavirus pandemic is currently the most important problem in the country and worldwide or did not provide their age were excluded from the analysis. This resulted in a total sample of 306 participants (229 women) that were used in the data analysis.

Pearson's coefficient was used to examine the intercorrelations of the Basic Hope, Meaning in Life, Satisfaction with Life, Anxiety, and COVID-19 Stress scales as well as gender and age. Simple mediation analyses were conducted using *PROCESS* macro for SPSS 25 with gender and age as covariates. The indirect effects were computed using the bootstrap method of 5,000 samples with a 95% confidence interval. The indirect effect was deemed significant when the 95% confidence interval didn't cross zero. The estimates of the regression coefficients and indirect effects were completely standardized. The assumption of normality was examined using the Q-Q plots on the distribution of errors, for each mediation model separately. No serious deviations from the lines were found.

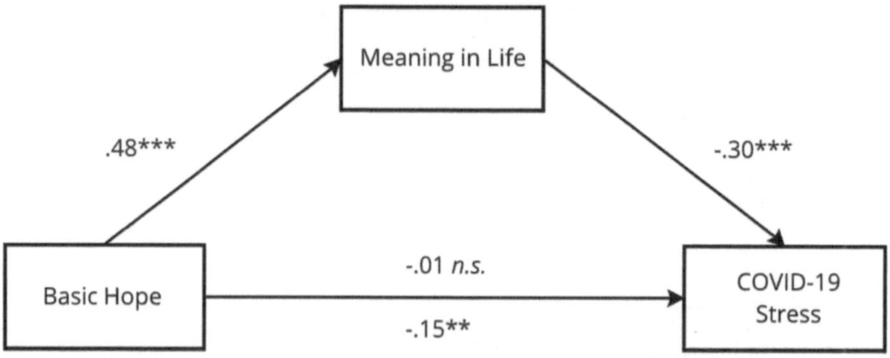

Figure 1. The model showing the mediating effect of Meaning in Life on the association between Basic Hope Total and COVID-19 Stress. *Note.* All coefficients were standardized. Gender and age were included as the covariates.

Correlations

Table 1 presents means, standard deviations, correlations, and—in the case of scales—Cronbach's alphas among gender, age, Basic Hope, Meaning in Life, Satisfaction with Life, State Anxiety (STAI), and COVID-19 Stress. The results show that Anxiety was positively associated with Reaction to Coronavirus and both were negatively related to Basic Hope, Meaning in Life, and Satisfaction with Life, although COVID-19 Stress was not significantly correlated with the Positivity subscale of Basic Hope. Satisfaction with Life, Meaning in Life, and Basic Hope were all positively correlated. From the sociodemographic variables, being a female was associated with a higher Anxiety and COVID-19 Stress, while age was positively related to Basic Hope—total and positivity subscale—Meaning in Life, and Satisfaction with Life.

Mediation analyses

Figures 1–4 show the analyzed mediation models. The two estimates that represent the relationship between the predictor and dependent variable are direct effect (upper) and total effect (lower). As discussed, each model was controlled for gender and age.

Basic Hope Total was positively associated with Meaning in Life ($\beta = 0.481$; $p < .001$) and the latter was negatively associated with COVID-19 Stress ($\beta = -0.30$; $p < .001$). Meaning in Life significantly mediated the effect of Basic Hope on COVID-19 Stress, BCa CI 95% [-0.23; −0.07]. Since the direct effect was not significant ($\beta = -0.010$; $p = .879$), there was a complete mediation effect.

Figure 2 shows that Basic Hope Total was positively related to Satisfaction with Life ($\beta = 0.386$; $p < .001$). Satisfaction with Life was, in turn, negatively correlated with Reaction to Coronavirus ($\beta = -0.195$;

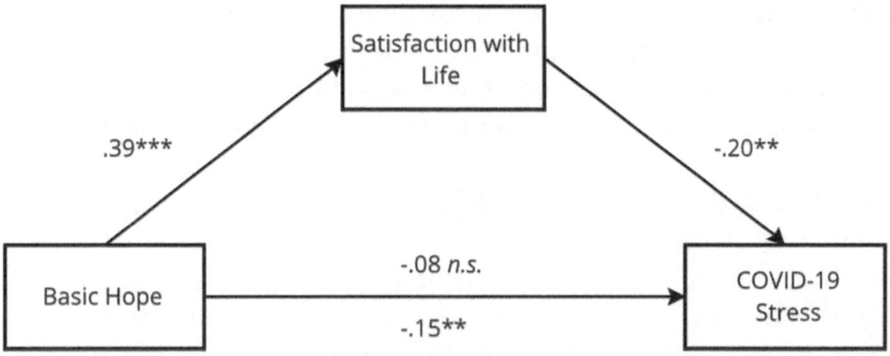

Figure 2. The model showing the mediating effect of the Satisfaction with Life Scale on the association between Basic Hope Total and COVID-19 Stress. *Note.* All coefficients were standardized. Gender and age were included as the covariates.

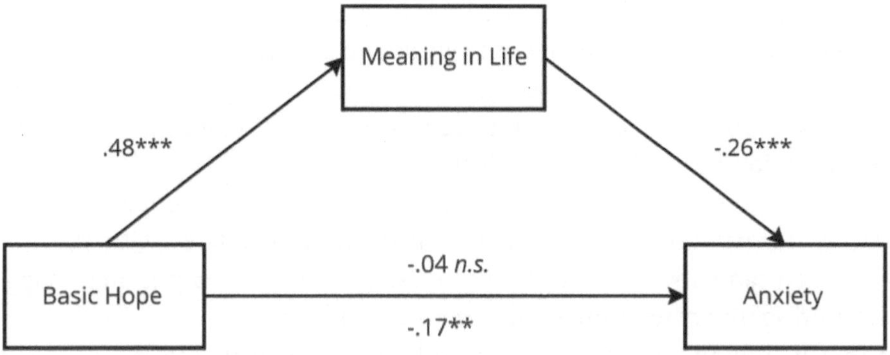

Figure 3. The model showing the mediating effect of Meaning in Life on the association between Basic Hope Total and Anxiety. *Note.* All coefficients were standardized. Gender and Age were included as the covariates.

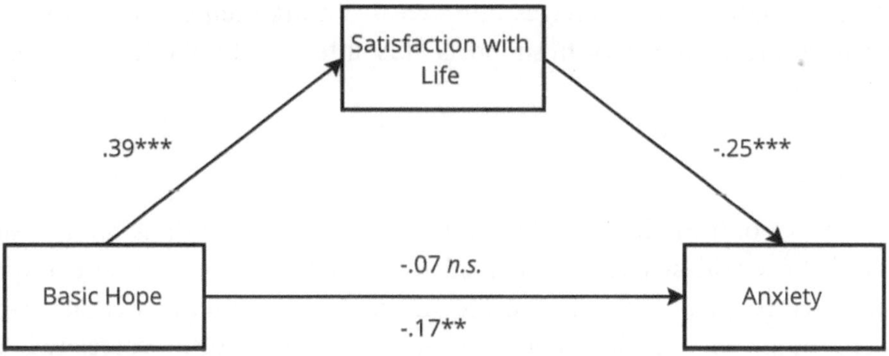

Figure 4. Model showing the mediating effect of Satisfaction with Life Scale on the association between Basic Hope Total and Anxiety. *Note.* All coefficients were standardized. Gender and Age were included as the covariates.

$p = .001$). There was a significant mediating effect of Satisfaction with Life on the relationship between the Basic Hope and COVID-19 Stress, BCa CI 95% [−0.13; −0.03]. The direct effect was found to be not significant ($\beta = -0.078$; $p = .195$) which means that there was a complete mediation effect.

Mediation analysis displayed in Figure 3 revealed that Basic Hope Total was positively associated with Meaning in Life ($\beta = 0.481$; $p < .001$) and the latter was, in turn, negatively associated with Anxiety ($\beta = -0.263$; $p < .001$). Meaning in Life significantly mediated the effect of Basic Hope on Anxiety, BCa CI 95% [−0.20; −0.06]. As the direct effect was not significant ($\beta = -0.039$; $p = .537$), the mediation effect can be said to be complete.

Finally, as Figure 4 shows, Basic Hope Total was positively correlated with Satisfaction with Life Scale ($\beta = 0.386$; $p < .001$). Further, Satisfaction with Life was negatively associated with Anxiety ($\beta = -0.254$; $p < .001$). The mediating effect of Satisfaction with Life on the relationship between the Basic Hope and Anxiety was deemed significant, BCa CI 95% [−0.16; −0.05]. The direct effect was not significant ($\beta = -0.067$; $p = .261$), thus there was a complete mediation effect.

Overall, the analyses indicate that the strength of basic hope and higher levels of the meaning in life and life satisfaction correlates with the lower state anxiety and lower COVID-19 stress. Mediation analysis may suggest the following interpretation of the interdependencies: basic hope supports meaning in life and life satisfaction and the increase in the latter two factors results in lower anxiety and COVID-19 stress. The mediation findings are in line with our expectations. It is worth noting that data from other experiments indicate that time orderliness in everyday activity and orderliness in simple perceptual images reinforce—although temporarily—the person's meaning in life, which supports this interpretation (Heintzelman & King, 2019).

Discussion

The results confirm the expectation that general assumptions about one's life and the world at large are related to a reaction to sudden and unpredictable danger. High meaning in life and life satisfaction, as well as strong presumptions on orderliness and positivity of the world, correlate with fewer panic thoughts and emotions evoked by the apparent danger of the ongoing CONVID-19 pandemic.

We expected that these three factors would appear important, especially when there are opportunities to reflect on the ongoing situation. Reflection allows considerate deliberation of the meaning and consequences of the danger and a person's judgments on the self and the world might become important then. The ongoing COVID-19 pandemic, at least at present and at least among ordinary people, should limit reflective thinking on the emergent situation. The danger is too direct, fast-paced, and unpredictable; furthermore, it has a massive, worldwide character. Our attention, thoughts, and emotions are under the control of direct signals of the danger, provided mostly by daily images and facts seen in mass media. Very often, these signals quickly evoke fear reactions and facilitate catastrophic associations and thoughts leading to the tendency to create and ruminate on the worst possible scenarios. The strong connection between state anxiety and intensity of negative thoughts activated by the pandemic makes the occurrence of a self-reinforcing spiral of emotions and thoughts likely. Surely, there is no optimal time to reflect on the present state and especially on the future consequences of the pandemic. Nevertheless, although the correlations are not high, the results of the study indicate that even in such circumstances a person's high meaning in life, life satisfaction, and the basic hope act as a buffer against the panic reactions on the virus pandemic. In line with the expectation, stronger assumptions of the world's orderliness and positivity influence reaction to the pandemic indirectly, by the mediation of meaning in life and life satisfaction. This buffer is important, if not dominant, in a person's reactions to the COVID-19 pandemic. It doesn't suppress the concern about the pandemic or openness to the relevant messages. However, it provides the background to a more rational and deliberative attitude and coping strategies toward the event.

Panic is counter-productive. Self-reinforcing spirals of anxiety and emotional reactions to the pandemic may result in nonrational behaviors and decisions that can even be self-destructive, especially when they have long-term consequences. For example, prolonged negative strong emotions disrupt social bonds. The three studied factors facilitate the stop-to think attitude when faced with threatening events.

In our model, basic hope, meaning in life, and life satisfaction are stable factors that influence thoughts and emotions in case of mortal danger. However, if the danger is prolonged and it disrupts the life order, the evoked thought and evaluations of the future and the present situation my steadily change all three factors. This could be due to the synergy effect: situational factors (ongoing danger) and their direct interpretation change basic assumptions which in return influence the interpretation of the ongoing danger circumstances. Several studies suggest that the strength of basic hope might be broken, at least temporarily, by important negative experiences such as exclusion or inclusion by an important social group (Abrams et al., 2005); a breakdown of long, intimate, and important relationship (Franklin et al., 1990; Janoff-Bulman, 1992); social anomie (Durkheim, 1952); and instability of social rules, high mortality, and poverty in macro-social environments (Griskevicius et al., 2011; Simpson et al. 2012 Worthman & Kuzara, 2005).

An unpredictable social environment, together with resource scarcity, results in personal life strategies, such as a short-term time perspective, lack of investments in the future for oneself and one's children, and involvement in risky activity, that might be interpreted as a consequence of weak basic trust (Griskevicius et al., 2011). In fact, environmental unpredictability is a more accurate predictive factor for these strategies than the harshness of conditions. (Belsky et al., 2012; Brumbach et al., 2009; Simpson et al., 2012).

It is important to investigate the types of social experiences that in a time of danger and increasing virus panic might—even temporarily—consolidate a person's feelings of basic hope, meaning in life and life satisfaction. For example, how to situationally reinforce basic hope—a ground base for searching, planning, and plan execution and therefore the important buffer against panic reactions to the threat? We think that a sense of order might be regained even at the level of mundane personal life. Daily routines, regardless of adversities, may reinforce the meaning in life and world orderliness. Engagement in activities that are a part of one's routine is connected with higher meaningfulness of life (Heintzelman & King, 2019). Even simple perceptual experiences with ordered versus disordered sequences may have short term effects on meaning in life (Heintzelman & King, 2013). Higher time-structuring of daily activities has been connected with better mental health (Mckee-Ryan et al., 2005) and better well-being (Van Hoye & Lootens, 2013). The World Health Organization (WHO, 2020) advised ensuring routines and schedules for children, while it seems to be highly important for adults as well. The message is: let us keep the normality in our environment and routines. When old scripts and known events and scenes have been disrupted, let's find or create new ones.

Acts of altruistic help and sacrifice may reinforce belief in positive human nature. How much it is needed can be seen in spontaneous appreciation and calling medical staff "heroes" from the first days of the pandemic, broadly publicizing volunteer activities and acts of solidarity with them. People are moved and inspired by acts of will to help as performed by 99-year-old veteran Captain Tom Moore, who started walking lengths of his garden to raise money for UK medical services, and was met with enormous generosity of the Britons. There are numerous reports of ways of helping, even little ones: donating money for equipment for hospitals, volunteering to deliver meals to the seniors, psychologists organizing support free of cost and educating people to cope with the situation, nuns supporting residential care staff, music stars performing "Concert for the heroes" via the Internet from their homes for medical personnel. Altruism reinforces the "positivity" component of Basic Hope, that is the assumption that people are generally good and therefore I may get support or help when coping with evil and danger. Moreover, successes—even small ones—in helping others in unknown dangerous situations reinforce our assumption that the world—in general—is ordered and predictable and so controlled by us. This may confirm our convictions that our efforts will be rewarded with a happy ending.

References

Abrams, D., Hogg, M. A., & Marques, J. M. (Eds.). (2005). *The social psychology of inclusion and exclusion*. Psychology Press.

Antonovsky, A. (1987). *The Jossey-Bass social and behavioral science series and the Jossey-Bass health series. Unraveling the mystery of health: How people manage stress and stay well*. Jossey-Bass.

Batthyany, A., & Russo-Netzer P. (Eds.). (2014). *Meaning in Positive and Existential Psychology*. Springer. https://doi.org/10.1007/978-1-4939-0308-5.

Belsky, J., Schlomer, G. L., & Ellis, B. J. (2012). Beyond cumulative risk: Distinguishing harshness and unpredictability as determinants of parenting and early life history strategy. *Developmental Psychology*, *48*(3), 662–673. https://doi.org/10.1037/a0025837.

Bowlby, J. (1986). *Attachment. Attachment and Loss* (vol. 1, 2nd ed.). Basic Books.

Bowlby, J., & Ainsworth, M. D. S. (1965). *Child care and the growth of love* (2nd ed.). Penguin Books.

Bretherton, I. (1992). The origins of attachment theory: John Bowlby and Mary Ainsworth. *Developmental Psychology*, *28*(5), 759–775. https://doi.org/10.1037/0012-1649.28.5.759.

Brumbach, B. H., Figueredo, A. J., & Ellis, B. J. (2009). Effects of harsh and unpredictable environments in adolescence on development of life history strategies: A longitudinal test of an evolutionary model. *Human Nature, 20*(1), 25–51. https://doi.org/10.1007/s12110-009-9059-3.

Diener, E., & Biswas-Diener, R. (2008). *Happiness: Unlocking the mysteries of psychological wealth.* Blackwell Publishing. https://doi.org/10.1002/9781444305159

Diener, E., Emmons, R. A., Larsen, R. J., & Griffin, S. (1985). The satisfaction with life scale. *Journal of Personality Assessment, 49*(1), 71–75. https://doi.org/10.1207/s15327752jpa4901_13.

Durkheim, É. (1952). *Suicide: A Study in Sociology.* Routledge & Kegan Paul.

Erikson, E. H. (1968). *Identity, youth and crisis.* W. W. Norton Company.

Franklin, K. M., Janoff-Bulman, R., & Roberts, J. E. (1990). Long-term impact of parental divorce on optimism and trust: Changes in general assumptions or narrow beliefs? *Journal of Personality and Social Psychology, 59*(4), 743–755. https://doi.org/10.1037/0022-3514.59.4.743.

Griskevicius, V., Tybur, J. M., Delton, A. W., & Robertson, T. E. (2011). The influence of mortality and socioeconomic status on risk and delayed rewards: A life history theory approach. *Journal of Personality and Social Psychology, 100*(6), 1015–1026. https://doi.org/10.1037/a0022403.

Haidt, J. (2006). *The happiness hypothesis: Finding modern truth in ancient wisdom.* Basic Books.

Heintzelman & King (2013). Encounters with the objective coherence and the experience of the meaning in life. *Psychological Science 24*(6), 991–998. https://doi.org/10.1177/0956797612465878.

Heintzelman, S. J., & King, L. A. (2019). Routines and meaning in life. *Personality & Social Psychology Bulletin, 45*(5), 688–699. https://doi.org/10.1177/0146167218795133.

Hicks, J. A., & Routledge, C. (Eds.). (2013). *The experience of meaning in life: Classical perspectives, emerging themes, and controversies.* Springer Science + Business Media. https://doi.org/10.1007/978-94-007-6527-6.

Janoff-Bulman, R. (1992). *Shattered assumptions: Towards a new psychology of trauma.* Free Press.

Mckee-Ryan, F. M., Song, Z., Wanberg, C. R., & Kinicki, A. J. (2005). Psychological and physical well-being during unemployment: A meta-analytic study. *Journal of Applied Psychology, 90*(1), 53–76. https://doi.org/10.1037/0021-9010.90.1.53.

Report on COVID-19 in Poland 12th of April (2020). Center for the Study of Democracy, SWPS University.

Seligman, M. E. P. (1991). *Learned optimism.* A.A. Knopf.

Seligman, M. E. P. (2002). *Authentic happiness: Using the new positive psychology to realize your potential for lasting fulfillment.* Free Press.

Simpson, J. A., Griskevicius, V., Kuo, S. I.-C., Sung, S., & Collins, W. A. (2012). Evolution, stress, and sensitive periods: The influence of unpredictability in early versus late childhood on sex and risky behavior. *Developmental Psychology, 48*(3), 674–686. https://doi.org/10.1037/a0027293

Snyder, C. R., Cheavens, J., & Michael, S T. (1999). Hoping. In C. R. Snyder (Ed.), *Coping: The psychology of what works* (pp. 20–56). Oxford University Press.

Snyder, C. R., Sympson, S. C., Michael, S. T., & Cheavens, J. (2001). Optimism and hope constructs: Variants on a positive expectancy theme. In E. C. Chang (Ed.), *Optimism & pessimism: Implications for theory, research, and practice.* (pp. 101–125). American Psychological Association.

Spielberger, C. D. (1983). *Manual for the State-Trait Anxiety Inventory* (rev. ed). Consulting Psychologists.

Steger, M. F., Frazier, P., Oishi, S., & Kaler, M. (2006). The meaning in life questionnaire: Assessing the presence of and search for meaning in life. *Journal of Counseling Psychology*, *53*(1), 80–93. https://doi.org/10.1037/0022-0167.53.1.80.

Trzebiński, J., & Zięba, M. (2004). Basic hope as a world-view: An outline of a concept. *Polish Psychological Bulletin*, *35*(3), 173–182.

Trzebiński, J., & Zięba, M. (2013). Basic trust and posttraumatic growth in oncology patients. *Journal of Loss and Trauma*, *18*(3), 195–209. https://doi.org/10.1080/15325024.2012.687289.

Van Hoye, G., & Lootens, H. (2013). Coping with unemployment: Personality, role demands, and time structure. *Journal of Vocational Behavior*, *82*(2), 85–95. https://doi.org/10.1016/j.jvb.2013.01.004

WHO. (2020, April 10). *Helping children cope with stress during the 2019-nCoV outbreak*. https://www.who.int/docs/default-source/coronaviruse/helping-children-cope-with-stress-print.pdf?sfvrsn=f3a063ff_2.

Worthman, C. M., & Kuzara, J. (2005). Life history and the early origins of health differentials. *American Journal of Human Biology: The Official Journal of the Human Biology Council*, *17*(1), 95–112. https://doi.org/10.1002/ajhb.20096

Zięba, M., Czarnecka-van Luijken, J., & Wawrzyniak, M. (2010). Nadzieja podstawowa i wzrost potraumatyczny [Basic hope and posttraumatic growth]. *Studia Psychologiczne*, *49*(1), 109–121.

Zięba, M., Surawska, M., & Zalewska, A. M. (2018). Relationships between personality traits, general self-efficacy, self-esteem, subjective well-being, and entrepreneurial activity. *Polish Psychological Bulletin*, *49*(2), 131–140. https://doi.org/10.24425/119480

Longing for a Familiar Way of Going Forward

Peter Joseph Gloviczki

ABSTRACT
This essay uses autoethnographic exploration to examine the lived experience of the COVID 19 virus. I particularly consider our transnational moment, with new platforms of/for work, and work to confront a sense of longing for a familiar way of going forward.

Today is March 18, 2020. I woke up this morning to an actual fog outside. Fitting, amidst the COVID 19 virus, how it is pressing us to reconsider what we know to be clear. Longing for clarity, I reach for the poet Paul Guest. Guest writes, in a poem for Eliot Khalil Wilson called "My Luck": "My best friend toils in a land/named Minnesota where sunlight is also optional" (Guest, 2008, p. 78). This line resonates with me in a variety of ways. I know Eliot as a man who was my teacher. I know Paul through his work. I know Minnesota as the land of my youth. I know sunlight there is either warm (in the summer) or cold (in the winter). I am longing, amidst COVID 19, for clarity in conditions, in weather, in any(every)thing.

With the daily development of the virus, I wonder where we will be in one week. I had been looking forward to traveling today. Postponed for now, in the way the best place for anyone to be amidst our transnational moment is inside. And so I put my courses online, posted videos and audios and wrote emails and sent/send them. Author(ed) daily emails. Connected/ting with my students virtually, through digital tools. The impact is still in development, yet to unfold. Philosopher Hubert L. Dreyfus asserts: "learning by apprenticeship can work only in the nearness of the classroom and laboratory; never in cyberspace" (Dreyfus, 2003, p. 583). I wonder, if not worry, if Dreyfus might be right in an emergency. The pace with which we all brought everything online. And yet we taught seminars and gave workshops. We held drop-ins and shared beverages and stories. Were we not as prepared as we could have been? I think we were. I wonder, as always, how I might have done more?

Ever the optimist, I read my students' work, interact with them, from home. I lean toward "what can be counted as real in virtual space" (Turkle, 1995, p. 323). I remind them all in various ways that it is okay, even expected, to feel stress, loneliness, disconnection from the routine, in these difficult times. The autoethnographer (Ellis & Bochner, 2000) always interplays self and other (Reed-Danahay, 1997). The interplay is today more concretely defined, owing to COVID 19: the self is at my home here, the other is at their home there. To me, boundaries are uncomfortably finite in an emergency. I look for ways to permeate boundaries. I continue my daily routines. Treadmill, pushups, texting. I stay mostly indoors. I take reasonable steps to try and follow the guidance. I wait for my work to reopen, to reunite with students so that we might continue our lessons. Is COVID 19 our new normal? I hope not. I am longing for clarity, for what was normal: a familiar way of going forward.

References

Dreyfus, H. L. (2003). Anonymity versus commitment: The dangers of education on the internet. In R. C. Scharff & V. Dusek (Eds.), *Philosophy of technology: The technological condition* (1st ed., pp. 578–584).Blackwell.

Ellis, C., & Bochner, A. P. (2000). Autoethnography, personal narrative, reflexivity. In N. K. Denzin & Y. S. Lincoln (Eds.), *Handbook of qualitative research* (2nd ed., pp. 733–768). Sage.

Guest, P. (2008). *My index of slightly horrifying knowledge.* Ecco/HarperCollins.

Reed-Danahay, D. (1997). *Auto/ethnography: Rewriting the self and the social.* Berg.

Turkle, S. (1995). *Life on the screen: Identity in the Age of the Internet.* Simon and Schuster.

The COVID-19 Pandemic Crisis: The Loss and Trauma Event of Our Time

Eric D. Miller

ABSTRACT
This paper provides the author's assessment of the nature of the coronavirus (COVID-19) pandemic crisis as of the period from mid-March to mid-April 2020. This analysis at this early stage of this crisis does not aim to offer specific predictions regarding how this emergency will continue to evolve or ultimately end. Instead, it documents key themes and issues that have developed during the earliest phase of the crisis and it utilizes known select points from the preexisting scientific literature in order to provide insight into some of the core issues that psychologists and other social scientists (in particular) will likely strive to investigate in the coming months and years. Issues involving loss, mental health, prosocial and destructive social behavior, and social, economic, and political matters are particularly highlighted.

At the time of this writing, the complete effects of the coronavirus pandemic that emanated in China in late 2019 were far from clear. In a March 12, 2020 *Wall Street Journal* editorial, Peggy Noonan, the famed speechwriter to former President Ronald Reagan, wrote:

> Now it's time to lose the two most famous phrases of the moment. One is "Don't panic!" The other is "an abundance of caution"… "Don't panic," in the current atmosphere, is a way of shutting up people who are using their imaginations as a protective tool. It's an implication of cowardice by cowards. As for "abundance of caution," at this point, in a world-wide crisis, the cautions we must take aren't abundant, they're reasonable and realistic. Reason and realism are good. (Noonan, 2020)

With this quote duly noted, this paper merely reflects the author's assessment of this crisis as of mid-March to mid-April 2020. While this paper does not attempt to proffer any absolute predictions about how this crisis will continue to evolve or end, it does try to utilize known evidence and scientific literature in order to provide an overview of how this crisis has evolved in its earliest stages and a possible roadmap of sorts for issues that psychologists and other social scientists (in particular) will likely want and need to assess in the coming months and years.

The coming months—and years

A March 20, 2020 *New York Times* analysis featured an assortment of opinions from eminent epidemiologists regarding the most plausible best and worst case scenarios for how the coronavirus pandemic will end with a particularly devastating worst case scenario of over 2 million dead in the United States (Kristof, 2020). Part of this analysis includes the rather likely scenario that countless Americans will die of other non-COVID-19 health conditions (such as heart disease and cancer) in the coming months (or even years) because they were unable or apprehensive about receiving proper medical treatments. In the best case scenario, the virus mutates, and helped with the warm summer 2020 months—coupled with additional newly-found therapeutic interventions—its effects are not as devastating as feared. Part of this scenario includes more of the aggressive social distancing measures and mass testing that proved to be especially beneficial to China and South Korea, in curtailing the number of cases in these respective countries. Of note, to date, the United States has not been fully able or willing to utilize these practices—and, if anything, the Trump administration has voiced frustration over the adverse economic impacts of mass business closures with a hope of possibly reducing these restrictions (Alexander & Pettypiece, 2020) even while there is growing scientific evidence that the virus is incredibly contagious and strong social distancing is necessary to prevent its transmission (Sanche et al., 2020). Indeed, a lasting legacy of the early stages of this crisis will be its checkered piecemeal response from governmental officials at federal, state, and local levels such as the frenzied rush to accumulate medical supplies like ventilators (Yong, 2020). Though there has been first a 15-day and then a 30-day "Stop the Spread" guideline from the White House, no national stay-at-home order was ever issued. And while the overwhelming majority of States did provide such guidelines they were often done in haphazard ways, such as New York City's initially lax decision to shut public schools or parks or Florida's similarly nonchalant attitude about closing its beaches during the height of the college Spring Break season where many of the young attendees offered like attitudes such as "If I get corona, I get corona" (O'Kane, 2020a).

By mid-April 2020, Dr. Anthony Fauci, a leading immunologist and key member of the White House Coronavirus Task Force, suggested that the total death toll may be less than initially feared where the deaths may perhaps only be in the tens of thousands rather than the hundreds of thousands or more (Chappell, 2020)—though he has also conceded that this virus could become endemic (Fauci et al., 2020). Given that this is a rapidly evolving situation as of this writing, not only is it impossible to predict the final death toll of this pandemic but also there is so much about the nature and effects of the COVID-19 disease that currently largely remains unclear or unknown. Epidemiologist Greta Bauer (2020) nicely summarizes the following key points: it is not clear whether immunity is certain after an infection or whether reinfection is possible, the long-term effects (such as, but not limited to the heart and lungs) are unknown, and though those who contract this virus are likely to survive it—many, including the young, will experience serious symptoms or even require hospitalization.

Real and potential loss and mental health challenges

At the time of this writing in mid-April 2020, the United States death toll stands at over 30,000, which eclipses the losses experienced due to the September 11, 2001 terrorist attacks ten-fold and growing. In what seems like a cruel irony, at least in the initial stages of this crisis, New York City and its greater metropolitan area are disproportionately represented in these statistics. Psychologists have long understood that data can be interpreted in different ways depending on how it is framed (Tversky & Kahneman, 1981). For instance, in the year 2017 alone, around 650,000 Americans died from diseases of the heart, which has long been the leading cause of death in the United States (Heron, 2019). But, we do have ways to reasonably prevent and treat conditions like cardiovascular disease which is not currently the case for COVID-19. Once more, at the time of this writing, the ultimate final death toll of the pandemic is yet to be determined and it is unclear how that final number will impact how individuals respond to and reflect on the pandemic and its impact for oneself and society. But, if we are to consider the COVID-19 pandemic as an event, it seems very plausible to reason that the final American death toll will eclipse the approximate 58,000 causalities from the Vietnam War; and, of course, this event had a profound impact on American society (Kieran, 2014). From there, only the American causalities associated with World War I, World War II, the Civil War, or the 1918 pandemic have amassed greater death tolls and, here again, all of these events profoundly reshaped United States and world history.

The experience of death tends to have personal and interpersonal components. A significant part of what has made this pandemic so disturbing are the number of cases where individuals were unable to be with or say goodbye to their loved one—or, if they were relatively fortunate enough, to do so via telephone or cellphone—as they were dying due to fears of transmission of the virus (Burke, 2020). This grief was likely compounded by the fact that, in many instances, family members were unable to hold burial services per their wishes (Kramer, 2020). COVID-19 is a disease that, thus far, has particularly prayed on the most vulnerable in our society—the elderly and those with preexisting health conditions such as heart or lung disease. Indeed, just as there have been shocking images emanating from hospitals (particularly in New York City) of both patients and corpses piling up, this has been true as well at many nursing home facilities (Leland et al., 2020). But, curiously, the ravages of this disease have not been limited to these aforesaid groups: Roughly 40% of all COVID-19 patients were under the age of 50 and there have been many cases of seemingly healthy younger adults (and some select minors) who have succumbed to this disease (Pinsker, 2020). COVID-19 has again shown the inequalities of our health care system in that minorities, particularly African-Americans, have had disproportionately higher death rates likely due to higher rates of preexisting medical conditions which have very clear linkages to health care disparities in the United States (Chappell, 2020).

Psychologists and other scholars have long noted humans' ability to survive and adapt with serious change and adversity. This was shown in the aftermath of the September 11, 2001 attacks where there were heightened levels of distress soon after the attacks but such symptoms tended to subside in the subsequent months (e.g., Neria et al., 2011). But, these terrorist attacks represented a singular event rather than a prolonged crisis which will likely define this pandemic; and, indeed, we know that prolonged stressors can be particularly difficult to adapt to (Walter, 2020). But, here too, we can take refuge in historical research and evidence that, even in the midst of war, people do find a way to function and survive such as when Londoners managed to periodically leave their underground bunkers to gather supplies in between German bombings during World War II (Field, 2002). In fact, a key tenet of adaptation level theory is that though major seemingly positive or negative events can at least have some marked short-term changes in mood, these appraisals tend to subside with time such that individuals tend to resort to their general outlook before the event (Brickman et al., 1978). Indeed, psychologists have long emphasized that it is not events per se that have the greatest impact on coping but rather how we perceive and ascribe meaning to them (e.g., Harvey & Miller, 1998). Likewise, psychologists have long found that those at greatest risk for psychopathology and more serious psychological symptoms tend to be those who were more likely have such symptoms before a given loss or trauma event (Wortman & Silver, 1989). We already know that those with preexisting psychological problems, such as anxiety, are already facing difficulties in adjusting to the realities and fears of the pandemic (Wiederhold, 2020). It is also known that disasters and crises can tax interpersonal relationships particularly those that were already distressed prior to the trauma (Harvey et al., 1995). And, there is already evidence of increased reports of domestic violence and abuse in the wake of the pandemic with its greater emphasis on staying at home (Campbell, in press). In sum, it is indeed quite possible that this crisis will directly or indirectly create or exacerbate personal and interpersonal crises.

This analysis is not to suggest that there may still yet to be far-reaching psychological effects on others emanating from this pandemic. We may yet to see spikes of suicides among individuals who cannot cope with the (actual or perceived) realities of the crisis (Reger et al., 2020). There will likely be heightened spikes of post-traumatic stress amongst those who have become seriously ill or have lost others (Pinsker, 2020). Medical personnel, first responders and other essential workers (including grocery workers) who have been on the frontlines may have unique risks and burdens from this crisis as well; even among those who have had more limited personal impacts or effects, such individuals may feel vicarious or secondary trauma such as through repeated television or media coverage of the crisis (Faris, 2020). Yet, consistent with much of the loss and trauma literature, we can find positive and meaningful ways to cope with this crisis through proven practices such as appreciating others and mindfulness (Polizzi et al., 2020).

Sometimes it just takes some time before individuals can truly understand how events impact them and they can do so in conflicting ways as depicted in some of the classic work by the late peace psychologist Milton Schwebel. In studying some of the immediate effects of the Cold War and the Cuban Missile Crisis, in particular, Schwebel (1965) found no evidence of increased psychopathology amongst children and adolescents though they did show marked increases of concerns for the well-being of their families and friends as well as a concern for their own futures as well as that for civilization as a whole. Schwebel (1986) further added that the 1945 bombing of Hiroshima brought immediate joy to many at that time since it ushered a sense that World War II was finally coming to an end; but, these reactions soon shifted once it was it was clear how these weapons could have an overwhelming destructive impact on humans and the growing threat that such weapons now posed for humanity as whole. Perhaps out of heightened awareness of the real or potential consequences of catastrophe, we can take steps to learn from such events in order to prevent or minimize the occurrence of future calamities as what happened in the years following the 1918 pandemic (Barry, 2005).

The good, the bad, and the ugly of human behavior

Social psychologists have long showcased the potential of human behavior from compassion to destructive acts—and this crisis has proven to be no exception. The effects of disaster appear to be no different in that it can both destroy preexisting communities while also striving to build a sense of community and meaning (Walter, 2020). Much attention has also focused on more purely altruistic acts such the case of 25 year old Rebecca Mehra who responded to the cries of an elderly couple asking for her to shop in a supermarket due to their fear of being out in public (O'Kane, 2020b). In the earliest stages of the COVID-19 crisis, countless workers—from medical staff to food suppliers and cashiers—are helping to ensure the larger public good. Yet, these individuals—particularly medical workers—have been placed woefully at grievous risk of personal disease or death due to grotesque lack of personal protective equipment (or PPE). The debate over whether the American government has yet again—with the COVID-19 pandemic—experienced another 9/11 or Hurricane Katrina moment (Miller, 2006) in being largely negligent in anticipating or in initially responding to these crisis will likely continue for some time. But, the question over how the American health care system was left in such disarray—with, for instance, requiring medical personnel to have to wear garbage bags—is an issue that requires immediate and continued attention (Yong, 2020).

Other behaviors have shown even darker potentials of social behavior to varying degrees of noxiousness. Perhaps triggered by fears of a lack of food and supplies, many supermarket shelves have been routinely cleared (though usually replenished)—yet some items, such as cleaning supplies and toilet paper have been particularly difficult to obtain (and in some cases, there have been actual fights over these items between store patrons). In the case of toilet paper, many psychologists have focused on panic buying or feeling desperate to have control over primal needs but there are also legitimate supply chain issues as companies have had to reorient their demands toward home rather than business based products (Oremus, 2020). This point also reveals a larger societal fragility insomuch that most individuals are under a presumption that there will not be any further disruptions to utilities and technology. It is almost inevitable that other natural and manmade calamities will occur during this pandemic: From a sheer structural perspective, it is unclear how governmental authorities and the larger public will respond in the event of hurricanes, tornadoes, or mass shootings and the like (Macor, 2020). The latter suggestion highlights some of the particularly disturbing behavioral consequences of the pandemic. Previous groups have been incredibly stigmatized or shown bigotry in relation to disease outbreaks with perhaps the best known contemporary example being how gay men were initially treated in the wake of the HIV/AIDS epidemic in the 1980s (e.g., Herek & Glunt, 1988). Accordingly, Asian-Americans (regardless of their country of origin or nationality) have faced a great uptick in hate-related crimes (Tavernise & Oppel, 2020). There have also been cases of individuals who have even shown or threatened violence in the wake of the pandemic albeit for varying reasons such as fears of not maintaining proper social distancing (Sandoval, 2020) or a desire to purposely infect others with the virus (with such motives often rooted in hate; Sheth, 2020).

Social, economic, and political questions

A key practice that has been clearly shown to slow the transmission of spread of the virus is social distancing. Though this practice was widely (though not entirely) adopted in the United States in March and April 2020, it remains unclear for how long (and to what extent) this practice will need to remain in place; some estimates suggest that this practice could be necessary, to varying degrees, through the year 2022 (Kissler et al., 2020). To a very significant degree, we could examine the success of social distancing as an altruistic act of humanity insomuch that by complying with this act, it theoretically helps to protect others from contracting this virus; it remains to be seen how well individuals may respond to any future directives over even greater periods of time. However, as critical as a tactic as social distancing appears to be, this very act necessarily draws us further away from others (which may be particularly injurious to groups, such as the elderly and those with comorbid health risks) and, in turn, increase feelings of loneliness (Rokach, 2019). The use of social distancing raises some interesting questions about our trajectory of how we communicate and interact with others. Though there has been previous contradictory evidence to date as to whether such social media is beneficial to our psychological well-being (Miller, 2018) this crisis has seemingly accelerated our use of technology and social media to communicate with others and in ways that could be potentially beneficial (Wiederhold, 2020). Further, given some of the particularly grueling images emanating out of cities regarding this pandemic, while it remains to be seen how, if at all, urban life is permanently impacted by this crisis, there already are calls for architects, in particular, to reimagine designs that enhance well-being and health (Steele, 2020).

In order to allow for social distancing practices to be effective, most businesses and services not deemed to be "essential" (such as supermarkets, pharmacies, and select medical offices) were encouraged or effectively forced by governmental authorities to shutter. This action, not surprisingly, has led to unemployment rates largely not seen since the era of the Great Depression—and, indeed, it is widely speculated that the U.S. economy is likely headed to a severe recession if not a depression (Klein, 2020).

Historically, serious economic insecurity is not just associated with personal hardship but it also has a way of often producing unexpected and rather adverse future social and political events as well (Irwin, 2020). Indeed, there is also a well-documented body of research suggesting that awareness of personal loss and mortality often produces perceived threats against our worldview which can further produce insidious effects (Burke et al., 2010). Very few sectors have not been adversely impacted by this crisis. To highlight one brief example, both K-12 and higher education had to adapt to swiftly dismissing students from their respective schools and campuses in order to move to remote or online learning. For K-12 students, the inability to attend school poses additional strains on parents including food-based needs for their children. Both high school and college students (who had to quickly abandon their dorms) had to quickly readapt to an uncertain situation where their own futures (e.g., employment opportunities) were at least questionable and where many prospective graduates had to forego the traditional graduation ceremony (Andrew, 2020). And, teachers had to quickly readjust their curriculum and find ways to provide education to their students (although, at least in higher education, the ability to teach online has been increasingly realized for well over the past decade; Miller, 2014). Companies and institutions, such as schools and colleges, will likely continue to struggle to adapt to looming closures or social distancing requirements. As many have proffered, such as Dr. Anthony Fauci, there needs to be a regular assessment of the cost-benefit analysis of between deciding to close down aspects of the economy but ultimately prudent decisions for the greater public health should prevail (Alexander & Pettypiece, 2020).

In the context of this ongoing crisis, political questions almost seem of secondary concern. Yet, there have been cases where Americans have had to weigh their constitutional rights of voting with the health risks associated of possibility contracting or spreading the virus. Arguably, this dilemma took a particularly shocking turn when State Courts and even the U.S. Supreme Court allowed in person voting to occur on April 7, 2020 in Wisconsin for their primary during the height of the pandemic; the ironic image of an elected Republican Wisconsin leader declaring that in person voting was safe to do despite the fact he was covered in full body protective gear was not left unnoticed (Perano, 2020). The Wisconsin Primary notwithstanding, these images left many wondering and questioning how the 2020 Presidential campaign (including political conventions) and voting will occur with particular emphasis on the importance of absentee voting. Assuming that there are judicious and fair means of voting, the American electorate will, of course, render their verdict on their assessment of President Trump's handling of the COVID-19 crisis in November 2020.

Historians and political and social scientists will likely consider various questions as to how coronavirus may have shaped political considerations and vice-versa. For instance, Senator Bernie Sanders seemed primed to become the 2020 Democratic nominee just before the COVID-19 crisis became into focus and eventually hindered his ability to effectively campaign; if this crisis had not happened, would he have become the Democratic nominee instead of former Vice President Joe Biden? But, arguably, the larger question may be what governmental or social agencies may have failed to properly recognize, warn, and prepare the larger public for the looming threat of the pandemic? At the current time, there are serious questions about the possible culpability of the Chinese government and the World Health Organization (WHO) (Feldwisch-Brentrup, 2020) as well as the Trump administration (Lipton et al., 2020). Another side issue to consider is how much the Trump administration may have been sidelined due to impeachment hearings that were underway right as the pandemic was ratcheting up in China. Ultimately, it may be most effective to review and learn from any such missteps so as to help recovery from this pandemic and to successfully anticipate, prevent, prepare, and address any subsequent ones.

Coda: A changed world?

Most psychologists realize the value and scientific importance of examining issues in as objective and dispassionate way as possible. Yet, scholars such as Ellis (2018) highlight the unique role and value of autoethnography where scholars are able to be "focusing outward on social and cultural aspects of their personal experience; then, they look inward, exposing a vulnerable self…" (p. 338). In this spirit, as I write this, I cannot help but to reflect on my own fears for myself and loved ones but also for our larger society. I wonder will I, or other members of my family, become ill—or so seriously ill to warrant hospitalization. I worry about my elderly mother who is living in New York City at the moment during this crisis. I have resigned myself to accepting that, at a minimum, I will likely know others whose health or lives have been grievously impacted by this virus.

Helen Branswell, a noted infectious diseases and public heath reporter, offered the following reflection in early March 2020:

> It's bizarre but I find myself startled. Having written about the possibility of something like this for years, I still find myself really startled that it's happening, and I don't know why that is. (Joseph, 2020)

I can relate to Branswell's sentiments insomuch that, as a social psychologist whose career has focused on how adults cope with adverse events and losses, I too share a sense of bewilderment that our world is experiencing this punishing pandemic. Then again, it is widely known that shock is a common reaction to highly stressful events—and professionals in the field are certainly not immune to such reactions (Walter, 2020).

Reflecting both my passion for psychology as well as history, I have often found it interesting how psychologists have covered seminal events and crises at the time they were occurring. It is widely known that World War II and the Holocaust spawned vast amounts of psychological research that helped reshape the field including (but not limited to) Milgram's legendary obedience studies; however, for a variety of reasons, there was a more muted response to its effects at the time while these events were going on and soon thereafter (Miller, 2017). Naturally, the field of psychology has evolved tremendously since then and careful attention has been examined to significant events that have impacted others and society such as the September 11, 2001 terrorist attacks (Silver, 2011). As a testament to the field, the response, effects, and consequences of the COVID-19 pandemic will certainly be examined by psychologists for decades to come. Perhaps this paper can help enlighten future students and scholars as to the immediate effects of the pandemic from what some have termed—as Winston Churchill famously put it—"the end of the beginning" of this crisis from the perspective of this psychologist.

References

Alexander, P., & Pettypiece, S. (2020, March 23). Tensions brewing inside the White House over economic consequences of coronavirus response. *NBC News*. https://www.nbcnews.com/politics/white-house/tensions-brewing-inside-white-house-over-economic-consequences-coronavirus-response-n1166671

Andrew, S. (2020, April 16). Why teens may never be the same after the pandemic. *CNN*. https://www.cnn.com/2020/04/16/us/teens-coronavirus-coping-wellness-trnd/index.html

Barry, J. M. (2005). *The great influenza: The epic story of the deadliest plague in history*. Penguin Books.

Bauer, G. (2020, April 8). Please, don't intentionally infect yourself. Signed, an epidemiologist. *The New York Times.* https://www.nytimes/com/2020/04/08/opinion/coronavirus-parties-herd-immunity.html

Brickman, P., Coates, D., & Janoff-Bulman, R. (1978). Lottery winners and accident victims: Is happiness relative? *Journal of Personality and Social Psychology, 36*(8), 917–927. https://doi.org/10.1037/0022-3514.36.8.917

Burke, B. L., Martens, A., & Faucher, E. H. (2010). Two decades of terror-management theory: A meta-analysis of mortality salience research. *Personality and Social Psychology Review, 14*(2), 155–195. https://doi.org/10.1177/1088868309352321

Burke, D. (2020, March 29). Coronavirus preys on what terrifies us: Dying alone. *CNN.* https://www.cnn.com/2020/03/29/world/funerals-dying-alone-coronavirus/index.html

Campbell, A. M. (in press). An increasing risk of family violence during the Covid-19 pandemic: Strengthening community collaborations to save lives. *Forensic Science International: Reports,* 100089. https://doi.org/10.1016/j.fsir.2020.100089

Chappell, B. (2020, April 9). Fauci says U.S. coronavirus deaths may be 'more like 60,000'; antibody tests on way. *NPR.* https://www.npr.org/2020/04/09/830664814/fauci-says-u-s-coronavirus-deaths-may-be-more-like-60-000-antibody-tests-on-way

Ellis, C. (2018). *Final negotiations: A story of love, loss, and chronic illness* (2nd ed.). Temple University Press.

Faris, D. (2020, March 19). Coronavirus' looming psychological crisis. *The Week.* https://theweek.com/articles/903343/coronavirus-looming-psychological-crisis

Fauci, A. S., Lane, H. C., & Redfield, R. R. (2020). Covid-19—Navigating the uncharted. *New England Journal of Medicine, 382*(13), 1268–1269. https://doi.org/10.1056/NEJMe2002387

Feldwisch-Brentrup, H. (2020, April 2). How WHO became China's coronavirus accomplice. *Foreign Policy.* https://foreignpolicy.com/2020/04/02/china-coronavirus-who-health-soft-power/

Field, G. (2002). Nights underground in darkest London: The Blitz, 1940–1941. *International Labor and Working-Class History, 62,* 11–49. https://doi.org/10.1017/S0147547902000194

Harvey, J. H., & Miller, E. D. (1998). Toward a psychology of loss. *Psychological Science, 9*(6), 429–434. https://doi.org/10.1111/1467-9280.00081

Harvey, J. H., Stein, S. K., Olsen, N., Roberts, R. J., Lutgendorf, S. K., & Ho, J. A. (1995). Narratives of loss and recovery from a natural disaster. *Journal of Social Behavior and Personality, 10,* 313–330.

Herek, G. M., & Glunt, E. K. (1988). An epidemic of stigma: Public reactions to AIDS. *American Psychologist, 43*(11), 886–891. https://doi.org/10,1037/0003-066X.43.11.886

Heron, M. (2019). Deaths: Leading causes for 2017. *National Vital Statistics Reports,* 68, 1–77.

Irwin, N. (2020, April 16). It's the end of the world economy as we know it. *New York Times.* https://www.nytimes.com/2020/04/16/upshot/world-economy-restructuring-coronavirus.html

Joseph, A. (2020, March 7). At Harvard forum, three who know warn of 'most daunting virus' in half a century. *STAT.* https://www.statnews.com/2020/03/07/harvard-forum-experts-warn-most-daunting-virus-in-50-years/

Kieran, D. (2014). *Forever Vietnam: How a divisive war changed American public memory.* University of Massachusetts Press.

Kissler, S. M., Tedijamto, C., Goldstein, E., Grad, Y. H., & Lipsitch, M. (2020). Projecting the transmission dynamics of SARS-CoV-2 through the postpandemic period. *Science,* eabb5793. https://doi.org/10.1126/science.abb5793

Klein, E. (2020, March 23). How the Covid-19 recession could become a depression. *Vox.* https://www.vox.com/2020/3/23/21188900/coronavirus-stock-market-recession-depression-trump-jobs-unemployment

Kramer, P. D. (2020, April 2). Burials without funerals, grief without hugs: Coronavirus is changing how we say goodbye. *USA Today.* https://www.usatoday.com/story/news/nation/2020/04/02/funerals-during-coronavirus-pandemic-no-hugs-big-gatherings/5102855002/

Kristof, N. (2020, March 20). The best-case outcome for the coronavirus, and the worst. *The New York Times.* https://www.nytimes.com/2020/03/20/opinion/sunday/coronavirus-outcomes.html

Leland, J., Harris, A. J., Tully, T. (2020, April 16). 29 Dead at one nursing home from the virus. Or more. No one will say. *The New York Times.* https://www.nytimes.com/2020/04/16/nyregion/new-york-nj-nursing-homes-coronavirus-deaths.html

Lipton, E., Sanger, D. E., Haberman, M., Shear, M. D., Mazzetti, M., Barnes, J. E. (2020, April 11). He could have seen what was coming: Behind Trump's failure on the virus. *The New York Times.* https://www.nytimes.com/2020/04/11/us/politics/coronavirus-trump-response.html

Macor, L. (2020, April 10). Florida's nightmare: A hurricane during the pandemic. *Yahoo! News.* https://news.yahoo.com/floridas-nightmare-hurricane-during-pandemic-012520230.html

Miller, E. D. (2006). Can Americans ever feel safe in a post-9/11 and Hurricane Katrina world?. In J. Forest (Ed.), *Homeland security: Protecting America's targets* (Vol. 2, pp. 350–364). Praeger.

Miller, E. D. (2014). The academic psychologist as a convener of information: Implications for the scholarship of integration and (online) teaching. *New Ideas in Psychology, 33,* 35–45. https://doi.org/10.1016/j.newideapsych.2014.01.001

Miller, E. D. (2017). Making sense of the brutality of the Holocaust: Critical themes and new perspectives. *The Journal of Psychology, 151*(1), 88–106. https://doi.org/10.1080/00223980.2016.1217191

Miller, E. D. (2018). Cyberloneliness: The curse of the cursor?. In O. Sagan & E. D. Miller (Eds.), *Narratives of loneliness: Multidisciplinary perspectives from the 21st century* (pp. 56–65). Routledge.

Neria, Y., DiGrande, L., & Adams, B. G. (2011). Posttraumatic stress disorder following the September 11, 2001, terrorist attacks: A review of the literature among highly exposed populations. *American Psychologist, 66*(6), 429–446. https://doi.org/10.1037/a0024791

Noonan, P. (2020, March 12). 'Don't panic' is rotten advice. *Wall Street Journal.* https://www.wsj.com/articles/dont-panic-is-rotten-advice-11584054431

O'Kane, C. (2020a, March 23). Florida college students test positive for coronavirus after going on spring break. *CBS News.* https://www.cbsnews.com/news/coronavirus-florida-spring-break-test-positive-covid-19-college-students-not-social-distancing-university-of-tampa/

O'Kane, C. (2020b, March 13). Woman helped elderly couple get food when they were too scared to go shopping during coronavirus outbreak. *CBS News.* https://www.cbsnews.com/news/coronavirus-elderly-rebecca-mehra-twitter-buys-couple-groceries-scared-to-go-into-store-during-oregon-outbreak/

Oremus, W. (2020). What everyone's getting wrong about the toilet paper shortage. *Marker.* https://marker.medium.com/what-everyones-getting-wrong-about-the-toilet-paper-shortage-c812e1358fe0

Perano, U. (2020, April 7). Wisconsin's GOP speaker defends holding election while draped in PPE. *Axios.* https://www.axios.com/Wisconsin-republican-speaker-election-coronavirus-dc08a298-2201-440a-9ef0-304f62ca570d.html

Pinsker, J. (2020, April 10). The pandemic will cleave American in two. *The Atlantic.* theatlantic.com/family/archive/2020/04/two-pandemics-us-coronavirus-inequality/609622/

Polizzi, C., Lynn, S. J., & Perry, A. (2020). Stress and coping in the time of COVID-19: Pathways to resilience and recovery. *Clinical Neuropsychiatry, 17*, 59–62. https://doi.org/10.36131/CN20200204

Reger, M. A., Stanley, I. H., & Joiner, T. E. (2020). Suicide mortality and coronavirus disease 2019—A perfect storm? *JAMA Psychiatry*, E1–E2. https://doi.org/10.1001/jamapsychiatry.2020.1060

Rokach, A. (2019). *The psychological journey to and from loneliness: Development, causes, and effects of social and emotional isolation.* Elsevier.

Sanche, S., Lin, Y. T., Xu, C., Romero-Severson, E., Hengartner, N., & Ke, R. (2020). High contagiousness and rapid spread of severe acute respiratory syndrome coronavirus 2. *Emerging Infectious Diseases, 26*(7). https://doi.org/10.3201/eid2607.200282

Sandoval, E. (2020, April 8). 86-Year-old is killed in E.R. over social distancing. *The New York Times.* https://www.nytimes/com/2020/04/08/nyregion/coronavirus-brooklyn-janie-marshall-cassandra-lundy.amp.html

Schwebel, M. (1986). The study of stress and coping in the nuclear age: A new specialty. *International Journal of Mental Health, 15*(1–3), 5–15. https://doi.org/10.1080/00207411.1986.11449016

Schwebel, M. (Ed.) (1965). *Behavioral science and human survival.* Science and Behavior Books. https://doi.org/10.1093/sw/10.4.119

Sheth, S. (2020, March 22). White supremacists discussed using the coronavirus as a bioweapon, explosive internal document reveals. *Business Insider.* https://www.businessinsider.com/coronavirus-white-supremacists-discussed-using-covid-19-as-bioweapon-2020-3

Silver, R. C. (2011). An introduction to "9/11: Ten years later". *American Psychologist, 66*(6), 427–428. https://doi.org/10.1037/a0024804

Steele, J. (2020, April 16). Architects forecast change for design in wake of COVID-19. *Forbes.* https://www.forbes.com/sites/jeffsteele/2020/04/16/architects-forecast-change-for-design-in-wake-of=covid-19/

Tavernise, S., & Oppel, R. A. Jr. (2020, March 24). Spit on, yelled at, attacked: Chinese-Americans fear for their safety. https://www.nytimes.com/2020/03/23/us/chinese-coronavirus-racist-attacks.html

Tversky, A., & Kahneman, D. (1981). The framing of decisions and the psychology of choice. *Science, 211*(4481), 453–458. https://doi.org/10.1126/sciemce.7455683

Walter, T. (2020). *Death in the modern world.* Sage.

Wiederhold, B. K. (2020). Using social media to our advantage: Alleviating anxiety during a pandemic. *Cyberpsychology, Behavior, and Social Networking, 23*(4), 197–198. https://doi.org/10.1089/cyber.2020.29180.bkw

Wortman, C. B., & Silver, R. C. (1989). The myths of coping with loss. *Journal of Consulting and Clinical Psychology, 57*(3), 349–357. https://doi.org/10.1037/0022-006X.57.3.349

Yong, E. (2020, March 25). How the pandemic will end. https://www.theatlantic.com/health/archive/2020/03/how-will-coronavirus-end/608719/

Philippine Teachers' Practices to Deal with Anxiety amid COVID-19

Karen Joy B. Talidong and Cathy Mae D. Toquero

ABSTRACT
School closures, home quarantine, and social distancing implemented worldwide can cause a sudden anxiety even among teachers. A designed online survey collected data from Filipino teachers' practices on how they deal with anxiety due to the COVID-19 outbreak. The practices include information seeking, preventive measures, and other coping mechanisms to deal with anxiety during the quarantine period. Results revealed that teachers practice virtual learning, communicate with the professional community, adhere to quarantine requirements, and find purposeful activities to deal with anxiety due to the suspension of national school-related activities in the country brought by the pandemic.

Introduction

When the Chinese government first announced the novel coronavirus outbreak in Wuhan, it was only days when it has been named as COVID-19 and eventually considered as a massive international concern. Such concern led the World Health Organization (WHO, 2020) to declare COVID-19 as a pandemic. In the Philippine context, when the imported and localized transmission of COVID-19 was recorded, the government considered it as a risk to national security (Nicomedes et al., 2020) (Nicomedes, Avila, & Arpia, 2020). Consequently, the Philippine government implemented the Enhanced Community Quarantine (ECQ) to contain the spread of COVID-19 on March 16, 2020. However, due to the increase of the COVID-19 cases in the Philippines, the ECQ was extended until April 30, 2020. This health problem created public health emergencies that Filipinos are also affected nationwide due to prolonged social isolation that creates loneliness, anxiety, depression, and can even lead to a post-traumatic stress disorder (Leite et al., 2020 cited American Psychological Society, 2020; WHO, 2020). The way of life in the Philippines has changed its course, although,

Filipinos are not the only ones whose life changed, considering that COVID-19 is already a global problem, everybody's lifestyle changed (Pan, 2020).

Considering the increase of COVID-19 cases in the Philippines, the researchers decided to find out the possible impact of COVID-19 outbreak to the people, particularly to the teachers on how they deal with the quarantine period. The Department of Education (DEPED) would have ended the school year for the basic level institutions in late March 2020, but due to COVID-19, the classes were shortened in the middle of the month. In case of an extension of the suspension of face to face education on the school year 2020–2021 due to the pandemic, the Department of Education launched the DEPED Commons Project to serve as an online platform for virtual lessons that teachers and even students nationwide can use as an alternative, but this is still on its trial stage and is not compulsory. Likewise, the Commission on Higher Education (CHED) also suspended the classes on the same month, but advised to deploy available distance learning and alternative modes, but which is not yet realized as of this moment since virtual learning is still new to the educational system in the Philippines.

Policies were created to secure the continuity of adherence of the stakeholders, particularly directed to the teachers and the students to the educational and preventive policies such as the provision of alternative delivery modes of education and quarantine requirements (Commission on Higher Education [CHED], 2020; Department of Education [DEPED], 2020). These new normal can posit worries to the teachers since they have not been trained for emergency online teaching. In addition, the suspension of classes even in higher education coupled with social isolation and home quarantine can cause anxieties to the teachers. Hence, both researchers decided to focus on an online survey about the experiences, attitudes, and practices of the teachers to deal with anxiety due to the COVID-19 pandemic.

Methods

Twenty-five questions were designed for an online survey about the practices, perceptions, and experiences of Filipino teachers on the COVID-19 outbreak. The respondents mostly came from Mindanao, Region XII, specifically in General Santos City, Sultan Kudarat Province, and South Cotabato Province. Teachers were chosen regardless of years of experience and institution level whether private or public employees. The teachers were asked for their voluntary participation in the study prior to the online administration of the instrument. The survey included seeking information, preventive measures, attitudes, psychological stress or anxiety, and practices to cope with their anxiety during the quarantine period. The online survey was disseminated from April 13 to April 16, 2020. After a week, 218 questionnaires were retrieved from the teachers. Data were analyzed using frequency and mean percentage a descriptive statistical treatment to interpret the teachers' responses.

Results and discussion

The teachers are not immune to the vulnerabilities due to COVID-19 since they had to discontinue teaching immediately after lockdown. However, they looked for ways to still communicate to families, colleagues, and a few of their students who are accessible online. Hereafter are the results of the teachers' practices to combat the effects of COVID-19.

In view of seeking information about COVID-19, 84.9% of Filipino teachers always search for news about the cases of COVID-19 per day and only 15.1% did not. On the other hand, 95.4% check the information about COVID-19 if it comes from a trusted or reliable source and a small portion of 4.6% do not care if what they are reading is reliable or not. With many speculations on COVID-19 and its negative impact on people, it is very important to be vigilant and careful with the news and information to believe. This is further reinforced by the WHO (2020) to seek information about COVID-19 once or twice a day, but they should be practical and only get information from trusted sources to plan and protect themselves and their loved ones.

In terms of the most important preventive measures to combat COVID-19, 44% of Filipino teachers consider avoiding crowded places, 6.4% of teachers suggest wearing face masks, 16.5% suggest washing hands, 20.2% observe proper hygiene, 2.7% take vitamins, 7.8% do exercise, stay at home at 1.4%, and there are two responses on following the government guidelines 0.9%. Moreover, 98.2% of Filipino teachers observe social distancing which is the highest percentage concerning the preventive measures to combat COVID-19. Part of the memorandum 019 of DEPED (2020) is to adopt information dissemination strategies and launch awareness campaigns about COVID-19 to prevent, control, and promote positive health behaviors and address fear and anxiety among the stakeholders. Likewise, Wilder-Smith and Freedman (2020) implied that social distancing helps to reduce the transmission of the virus. Social distancing is necessary for avoiding transmission of COVID-19, although it triggers a feeling of sadness and anxiety among people. The authors (Roy et al., 2020; Yang et al., 2020) suggest that it is important for people to be aware of the preventive measures to avoid transmission of COVID-19 through observing personal hygiene, using sanitizers, washing hands, and wearing masks. This also includes self-isolating, practicing social distancing, and drinking plenty of water (Roy et al., 2020).

Furthermore, 89% regularly check themselves for early symptoms of COVID-19, only 73.9% of Filipino teachers do not want to talk to some acquaintances without a mask, while 89% prefer to bring disinfectant alcohol with them when they go out. Likewise, there are 85.3% of teachers who disinfect their things before entering their house, 61% do not look forward to visiting public places like parks, and 57.8% do not look forward to spending some time with their friends like watching movies at malls.

Concerning the attitudes of the Filipino teachers during the quarantine period, 56% do not feel bored staying at home during quarantine, and only 44% feel otherwise. On the positive side, 93.1% feel positive spending time with their family during the quarantine. Given the activity that they always do during the quarantine period, 25.6% of Filipino teachers prefer watching television. Moreover, 23.8% of teachers prefer cooking and spending their time with other activities such as doing exercise (11.9%), sleeping (8.7%), playing mobile games (5.9%), writing (4.1%), gardening (5.9%), cleaning the house (3.2%), surfing the internet/Facebook (3.6%), praying (1.4%), reading (2.3%), and working with DepEd forms for checking (0.9%). Considering the results on the attitudes of the Filipino teachers during the quarantine period, teachers feel positive spending time with their families during the quarantine. This is a good preference among Filipinos as they give importance to their families. It has been in a Filipino culture that problems can be overcome having a family around. Likewise, it is necessary for the teachers to learn daily routines such as physical activities to reduce boredom and find ways to strengthen positive experiences to others. Keeping regular contact with loved ones through phone, social media, social networks, and creating new hobbies, and thinking positively can help alleviate anxiety amid the global crisis (WHO, 2020).

Because of the anxiety or psychological stress brought by COVID-19, 92.7% of Filipino teachers are not confident to go to crowded places, 91.3% do not feel secure with using public transportation, 89.9% are conscious in touching any surfaces at public areas, 79.3% are conscious to touch their faces without washing their hands, 81.7% have doubts in eating in a restaurant, 91.7% of Filipino teachers' lifestyle change because of the COVID-19, and 92.7% are afraid that their family members might be infected with COVID-19. The findings of this study show a positive outlook among Filipino teachers amid the COVID-19 pandemic, yet, psychological stress or anxiety is apparent in their lives. This is due to the fact that they are not able to do the things that they once used to do as their lifestyle changed during the pandemic (Pan, 2020).

For the ways to deal with anxiety during Enhanced Community Quarantine (ECQ), 74.8% of the Filipino teachers spend more time in social media, and, 78.8% discovered a new hobby while on quarantine. In addition, for the best way to cope with anxiety during COVID-19 outbreak, 53% of Filipino teachers prefer spending time with family, 30.2% seek spiritual guidance, 8.3% talk with friends online, and, 4.1% talk with their special someone online, while interestingly, a small portion of teachers, 1.8% talk to themselves. Finally, given the question, if their life will be back to normal when COVID-19 is over, 81.7% answered positively. As to the anxiety brought by COVID-19, Filipino teachers are hesitant to go to crowded places which are also supported by the perceived preventive measures for COVID-19 such as avoiding crowded places and social distancing. This statement supports the result of the study on the anxiety felt by the teachers amid the COVID-19 outbreak. To deal with anxiety, Filipino teachers have discovered a new hobby while on quarantine since most of them are also spending time with social media to communicate with friends, students, and colleagues and read news updates regarding COVID-19 since it can heighten their awareness during a crisis (Hocke-Mirzashvili et al., 2015). Likewise, teachers spend more time online since they also practice the virtual learning project aside from communicating through a professional online community with colleagues. They also developed ways to find something purposeful due to the suspension of all national and regional school-related conferences and activities in the country (CHED, 2020; DEPED, 2020).

Conclusion and implications

COVID-19 indeed changed the lives of many people around the world. It created fear, trauma, depression, and anxiety to people, especially those who lost their loved ones due to the pandemic. In the context of the Philippines, Filipinos, particularly the teachers are worried about the safety of their loved ones and even their lifestyles have been affected because of the fears due to the pandemic. Though the Filipino teachers have shown a positive outlook in life amid the COVID-19 outbreak, they are still susceptible to the anxieties since the pandemic is still ongoing worldwide. These teachers though are well aware of what to do to cope with their educational, social, and personal anxieties. Therefore, this article points out that there is ample evidence that the Filipino teachers practice measures to deal with anxiety since they adhere to the preventive and educational policies of DEPED and CHED in the fight against COVID-19. However, this study has its limitations such that it cannot be generalized to the entire teachers in the Philippines due to the limited number of teachers who answered the online survey, and this study mainly relied on self-reported experiences of the teachers. Nonetheless, the study presents social implications and novel value. The social implication of this study is grounded on the teachers' capability to communicate and follow the guidelines of the government for social distancing and other preventive measures as offered through social media. Likewise, this work has proven its originality since no studies are done prior to this that focus on the teachers' home quarantine experiences amid COVID-19. Further studies should be conducted that focus on the effectiveness of social media for communication purposes amid the health crisis and an in-depth investigation should be made that examines the effects of the pandemic to the emotional and mental well-being of the Filipino teachers including the population of the student community.

References

American Psychological Society. (2020). https://www.apa.org/practice/programs/dmhi/research-information/social-distancing.

Commision on Higher Education. (2020). *Memoranda about COVID-19.* https://ched.gov.ph/blog/2020/03/12/guidelines-for-the-prevention-control-and-mitigation-of-the-spread-of-the-2019-novel-coronavirus-acute-respiratory-disease-in-higher-education-institutions/

Department of Education. (2020). *Memoranda about COVID-19.* https://www.deped.gov.ph/covid-19/covid19-memoranda/

Hocke-Mirzashvili, T. M., Kelly, S., & MacDonald, P. (2015). Student evaluations of a university crisis communication response: The gunman threat at North Carolina A&T. *Public Relations Journal*, *9*(4), 1–24. http://www.prsa.org/Intelligence/PRJournal/Vol9/No4/

Leite, H., Hodgkinson, I. R., & Gruber, T. (2020). New development: 'Healing at a distance'—telemedicine and COVID-19. *Public Money & Management.* https://doi.org/10.1080/09540962.2020.1748855

Nicomedes, C. J., Avila, R. M., Arpia, H. M. (2020, April). The lived experiences of Filipino front liners during COVID-19 outbreak. https://www.researchgate.net/publication/340444633_The_Lived_Experiences_of_Filipino_Front_Liners_During_COVID-19_Outbreak

Pan, H. (2020). A glimpse of university students' family life amidst the COVID-19 virus. *Journal of Loss and Trauma*, 1–4. https://doi.org/10.1080/15325024.2020.1750194

Roy, D., Tripathy, S., Kar, S. K., Sharma, N., Verma, S. K., & Kaushal, V. (2020). Study of knowledge, attitude, anxiety, & perceived mental healthcare need in Indian population during COVID-19 pandemic. *Asian Journal of Psychiatry*, *51*, 102083–102087. https://doi.org/10.1016/j.ajp.2020.102083

Wilder-Smith, A., & Freedman, D. O. (2020). Isolation, quarantine, social distancing and community containment: Pivotal role for old-style public health measures in the novel coronavirus (2019-nCoV) outbreak. *Journal of Travel Medicine*, *27*(2), 1–4. https://doi.org/10.1093/jtm/taaa020

World Health Organization. (2020, March 18). Mental health and psychosocial considerations during the COVID-19 outbreak. https://www.who.int/docs/default-source/coronaviruse/mental-health-considerations.pdf

Yang, H., Bin, P., & He, A. J. (2020). Opinions from the epicenter: An online survey of university students in Wuhan amidst the COVID-19 outbreak1. *Journal of Chinese Governance*, 1–15. https://doi.org/10.1080/23812346.2020.1745411

Mental Health and Its Influencing Factors among Self-Isolating Ordinary Citizens during the Beginning Epidemic of COVID-19

Yuqing Zhao, Yuanyuan An, Xing Tan, and Xiaohui Li

ABSTRACT

The study aims to investigate the current prevalence of anxiety, depression and PTSD among self-isolating general population, mainly college students, in the context of COVID-19 from January 26, 2020 to February 2, 2020, and to provide guidance for the general public. A total of 515 self-isolating people completed the online questionnaire including questions asking for demographic information and the impact of COVID-19 on their (mental and physical) health. The results showed that prevalence of anxiety, depression and PTSD was 14.4, 29.7, and 5.6%, respectively. Given the high prevalent but poorly recognized psychological disorders among self-isolating population under COVID-19, suggestions are provided in enhancing the media management in hope to improve self-isolating people's understanding of the epidemic and themselves and, ultimately, the health and emotional well-being of the society.

Introduction

In December of 2019, Corona Virus Disease 2019 (COVID-19) first being identified in Wuhan province, quickly spread to other parts of China. As of right now, most of the countries in the world have infected cases reported. On January 30, 2020, the World Health Organization declared that the COVID-19 outbreak was a public health emergency of international concern (World Health Organization, 2020). The COVID-19 not only attacked the virus carriers' immune system jeopardizing their physical health rapidly, but also caused psychological harm to the general public in various degrees according to their exposure to panic media reports (Garfin et al., 2020; Qiu et al., 2020). Moreover, in attempt to restrain COVID-19, Wuhan went into lockdown on January 23, 2020; on January 26, 2020, the rest of China had been taking measures such as traffic control, prohibition of gathering, and social isolation as person to person transmissions were confirmed both inside and outside of China (CCTV News, 2020). Some recent published studies showed that people experienced self-isolation during the period of COVID-19 outbreak were more likely to develop symptoms of anxiety, depression and psychiatric disorders, such as post-traumatic stress disorder (PTSD) (Li et al., 2020; Liu, Chen, et al., 2020; Wang et al., 2020).

Anxiety is a kind of psychological stress accompanied by a series of physiological events and it could cause a decrease in immunity (Liu, Chen, et al., 2020). The general public's anxiety about COVID-19 is palpable because people are generally susceptible to it (Cui et al., 2019). In an interview with the self-isolating people, the results showed that 98.54% of the respondents were very scared of COVID-19 and 94.45% were anxious about whether they or their families would be infected (Qi et al., 2020). Anxiety and depression can co-occur in an individual (Zhong et al., 2020). A study reviewed existing literature about COVID-19 and suggested that 16–28% of the subjects screened reported depressive and anxiety symptoms (Rajkumar, 2020). An individual has his own psychological resources to deal with the stressor in his life, maintaining their mental health. While COVID-19 was new and unknown to everyone, people would feel little sense of control over this threat. Therefore, when people cannot properly deal with the feeling out of control caused by COVID-19 by using their existing psychological resources, they may develop symptoms of anxiety and depression (Mahmoud et al., 2012; Slovic & Peters, 2006).

PTSD is a delayed, long-term psychosocial syndrome that occurs after a person has suffered an overwhelming traumatic event (Khazaie et al., 2016). A study focusing on 285 residents of the most impacted region in China indicated that the prevalence of posttraumatic stress symptoms one month after the COVID-19 outbreak was 7% (Liu, Zhang, et al., 2020). It was obviously that the posttraumatic stress symptoms were common psychological responses appearing on people who underwent such kinds of public health emergencies. As to the self-isolating general population, they felt their lives were threatened because of the explosion of the mass information of COVID-19 and the invasion of COVID-19. Therefore, they were at high risk of developing PTSD symptoms. PTSD is a relatively serious psychological problem that affects individuals for a long time. These threatening psychological problems need early detection and intervention (An et al., 2019).

The mental health and psychological state of the self-isolating general population was particularly of our interest due to the following reasons: (1) COVID-19 was widely spread. The virus carriers or potential virus carriers were moving all around China with Spring Festival travel rush. COVID-19 can be transmitted from person to person, so people were aware that they can be infected and their lives were under threaten. (2) Since the outbreak of COVID-19, all kinds of media were propagating the information about the COVID-19, including rumors. This could cause mass panic. Researchers found that people with the highest exposure to media coverage of such kind of traumatic events had even more acute stress than people who were directly exposed to the trauma events (Giummarra et al., 2018).

This study aims to investigate the current status of anxiety, depression and PTSD among self-isolating general population (mainly college students) in the context of COVID-19, as well as the differences in the distribution of these factors in demographic variables, and to provide suggestions for self-protection.

Method

Participants

For this study, we recruited the participants from a group of self-isolating people in China, mainly college students, from January 26, 2020 to February 2, 2020. During this period, COVID-19 was identified and the information about COVID-19 was made public for a short time. Every day, the general public can receive an update on the exact number of patients, suspected cases, deaths and cures. A total of 515 participants completed the entire online questionnaire. 33.6% of participants were males and 66.4% were females. In terms of age, among all participants, 49.5% ($N = 134$) were less than 20, 38.4% ($N = 198$) were between 21 and 45, and 12% ($N = 62$) were over 45. As to provinces (cities) where they lived in the past six months, 39.2% ($N = 202$) of the participants had lived in Shandong of north China, 15% ($N = 77$) in Chongqing of southwest China, 23.7% ($N = 122$) in Jiangsu of east China, and the remaining 22.1% ($N = 114$) had lived in other parts of China. In terms of the provinces (city) where they were living when data were collected, 40% ($N = 206$) of the participants were in Shandong, 14.8% ($N = 76$) in Chongqing, 17.1% ($N = 88$) in Jiangsu, and the remaining 28.1% ($N = 145$) were living in other parts of China. 55.9% of the participants traveled to their hometown during the epidemic, and 44.1% of the participants were living in the same city as they were six months ago. Because the Chinese Spring Festival travel rush increased the possibility that general people being infected with COVID-19 made it important to understand the changes in their geographical location of them.

Procedure

The researchers sent the online questionnaire linked through "WeChat" App platform. The corresponding personnel in each region spread the news, recruiting self-isolating people who were willing to participate in the online survey to join the study from January 26, 2020 to February 2, 2020, when the measure of self-isolation were enforced (Gao, 2020). The sample of the study were able to grow as some of the participants voluntarily introduced the study to their friends and relatives through their own social media.The questionnaire used a uniform guide, which described the purpose of the survey, inclusion criteria and exclusion criteria. Once respondents agreed to participate in the survey, they can click on the start button to automatically jump to the formal questions of the survey. The participants were asked to complete the survey in a quiet place which allowed them to fill the questionnaires independently without interruption. After the survey was completed, the participants clicked submit, their answers to the questionnaires were automatically saved.

Measures

Sociodemographic information

Participants were asked to report their age, gender, residence for the past six months and present (province and city), and migration condition (whether went hometown while the Spring Festival) (yes vs. no). Here, people who were in migrate condition means people had lived in one city in the past 6 months and migrated to another city, maybe his hometown, during the Spring Festival. If people chose the same residence for the past six months and present, they were not in migrate condition; Otherwise, they were in migrate condition.

Self-Rating Anxiety Scale (SAS)

Anxiety was assessed by using the 20-item Self-Rating Anxiety Scale (Zung, 1971). The scale is scored at 4 points, with 1–4 representing “no or little time,” “a small amount of time,” “considerable time” and “most or all time” respectively. The original score multiplying by 1.25 after taking the integer part was counted as the standard score; the higher the standard score, the more obvious the symptoms were. According to the results of the Chinese norm, the SAS standard score is 50 points, among which 50–59 points are considered as mild depression, 60–69 points are considered as moderate depression, and 69 points or above are considered as major depression. In the current study, the scale had acceptable internal consistency reliability, with a Cronbach’s α of 0.63.

Self-Rating Depression Scale (SDS)

Depression was assessed by using the 20-item Self-Rating Depression Scale (Zung et al., 1965). The scale is scored at 4 points, with 1–4 representing "no or little time," "a small amount of time," "considerable time" and "most or all time," respectively. The original score was multiplied by 1.25 and the integral part was the standard score. The higher the standard score, the more obvious the symptoms were. According to the results of the Chinese norm, the SDS standard score is 53 points, among which 53–62 points are considered as mild depression, 63–72 points are considered as moderate depression, and 73 points or above are considered as major depression. In the current sample, consider that item 2, 5, 6, 11, 12, 14, 16, 17, 18, 20 were scored backwards, the scale had an acceptable internal consistency reliability, with a Cronbach's α of 0.64.

PTSD checklist for DSM-5(PCL-5)

PTSD was assessed by using the 20-item PTSD Checklist for DSM-5 (Blevins et al., 2015). The items were translated into Chinese by Zhou and colleagues (2018). The PCL-5 has four dimensions: (1) invasion, (2) avoidance, (3) emotion alteration, and (4) hyper-arousal. In this study, the respondents rated the frequencies of symptoms experienced after the start of COVID-19. Example items include "A sad thought or picture related to COVID-19, suddenly broke into my mind", "Trying to avoid activities, people or places that remind me of COVID-19", "I feel sad when I think of or listen to people talking about COVID-19 (e.g. feeling scared, angry, sad, and guilty, etc.)", "Over-alert (e.g. keep looking around people and environment to ensure safety)" for each dimension. The scale items were rated on a 4-point Likert scale ranging from 0 ("never") to 3 ("always"). Higher scores indicate more severe level of symptoms. According to the PTSD diagnostic criteria of DSM-5 (American Psychiatric Association, 2013), the following conditions were prevalence criteria for its dimension of invasion, avoidance, emotion alteration and hyper-arousal: (1) at least one item' score of the invasion subscale is equal to or more than 2; (2) at least one item' score of the avoidance subscale is equal to or more than 2; (3) at least two items' score of the emotion alteration subscale is equal to or more than 2; (4) at least two items' score of the hyper-arousal subscale is equal to or more than 2. Individuals who met all the above conditions were identified as having "high risk of suffering from PTSD." In the current sample, the scale had good internal consistency reliability, with a Cronbach's α of 0.90.

Data analysis

The data was analyzed using SPSS 23.0. We did the descriptive statistics, analysis of variance, and independent sample *T* test. There were no missing data in this study because each question in the online questionnaire

Table 1. Mean, standard deviation and prevalence of the variables and correlation among them.

Variable	M	SD	Prevalence	1	2	3	4	5	6	7
PTSD_invasion	3.510	2.526	47.8							
PTSD_avoidance	1.400	1.407	17.3	0.531***						
PTSD_emotion alteration	3.790	3.372	10.3	0.580***	0.415***					
PTSD_hyper-arousal	3.770	3.073	6.6	0.643***	0.410***	0.776***				
PTSD_total	12.470	8.739	5.6	0.824***	0.619***	0.893***	0.903***			
Depression	45.16	11.284	29.7	0. 335***	0.220***	0.510***	0.397***	0.469***		
Anxiety	39.010	9.259	14.4	0.371***	0.249***	0.505***	0.497***	0. 517***	0.594***	

Note: ***$p < 0.001$.

required participants to fill out to move to the next question. Harman's single factor test was used to examine common method bias (Podsakoff et al., 2003). The results showed that the variance explained by the first factor after not rotation and rotation respectively was 24.84 and 9.26%, which were both less than the critical value of 40%. Therefore, no signs for significant common method bias were detected in the current study.

Results

The mental health of self-isolating general population

As presented in Table 1, the mean score for anxiety, depression and PTSD were 39.01 ($SD = 9.26$), 45.16 ($SD = 11.28$) and 12.47 ($SD = 8.74$) for the participants of the study, respectively. Based on the criteria in measure, the prevalence of anxiety was 14.4%, and the prevalence of mild, moderate and severe anxiety were 11.5, 2.5, and 0.4%, respectively. The prevalence of depression was 29.7%, and the prevalence of mild, moderate and severe depression were 20.4, 8.5, and 0.8%, respectively. And the prevalence of PTSD among our participants was 5.6%, prevalence of invasion, avoidance, emotion alteration and hyper-arousal (the four dimensions of PTSD) were 47.8, 17.3, 10.3, and 6.6%, respectively.

The difference of mental health in age and migration condition

A comparison of the mental health of participants in different age groups indicated that participants' age matters in level of anxiety [F (515) = 5.56, $p < 0.01$]. The post hoc test results showed that the anxiety level of the participants older than 45 years old were significantly lower than those whose age was between 21 and 45 years old($ps < 0.01$), and those younger than 20 years old($ps < 0.001$). The prevalence rates of anxiety among participants younger than 20, between 20 and 45, and older than 45, were 14.1, 17.2, and 6.5%, respectively. Participants of different ages did not differ significantly in scores for depression and PTSD.

Table 2. Demographic differences in PTSD scores, depression scores, and anxiety scores ($N = 515$).

Variable	PTSD		Depression		Anxiety	
	M ± SD	t(F)	M ± SD	t(F)	M ± SD	t(F)
Age						
Total	12.47 ± 8.739	2.728	45. 16 ± 11.284	1.015	39.01 ± 9.259	5.561**
≤20	12.54 ± 7.826		45.69 ± 10.817		39. 54 ± 8.680	
21–45	13.10 ± 9.960		45.01 ± 11.694		39.46 ± 10.165	
>45	10.15 ± 7.834		43.45 ± 11.284		35.36 ± 7.720	
Gender						
Total	12.47 ± 8.739	0.446	45.16 ± 11.284	0.254	39.01 ± 9.259	1.157
Male	12.10 ± 9.561		44.80 ± 11.399		39.62 ± 10.473	
Female	12.65 ± 8.301		45.34 ± 11.238		38.70 ± 8.579	
Province (city) of residence for the past six months						
Total	12.47 ± 8.739	3.276*	45.16 ± 11.284	1.235	39.01 ± 9.259	4.201**
Shandong	11.31 ± 7.753		44.44 ± 11.090		37.77 ± 8.855	
Chongqing	12.19 ± 8.003		44.01 ± 9.774		38.20 ± 8.900	
Jiangsu	14.41 ± 10.308		46.53 ± 11.978		41.39 ± 9.963	
Others	12.62 ± 8.779		45.73 ± 11.762		39.20 ± 9.029	
Current province (city) of residence						
Total	12.47 ± 8.739	1.682	45.16 ± 11.284	0.443	39.01 ± 9.259	1.847
Shandong	11.70 ± 7.983		44.88 ± 10.947		38.14 ± 8.983	
Chongqing	12.33 ± 7.969		44.16 ± 9.748		38.32 ± 8.892	
Jiangsu	14.18 ± 9.616		45.67 ± 12.291		40.62 ± 10.201	
Others	12.59 ± 9.502		45.76 ± 11.915		39.61 ± 9.153	
Whether to go hometown						
Total	12.47 ± 8.739	0.869	45.16 ± 11.284	0.001	39.01 ± 9.259	1.289
Yes	12.78 ± 8.908		45.15 ± 11.225		39.42 ± 8.902	
No	12.06 ± 8.523		45.17 ± 11.383		38.49 ± 9.687	

Note: *$p < 0.05$, **$p < 0.01$.

A comparison of the mental health of participants with different migrate condition indicated that whether participants went hometown during the Spring Festival had an insignificant difference on anxiety [F (515) = 0.001, $p > 0.05$], depression [F (515) = 1.289, $p > 0.05$] and PTSD [F (515) = 0.869, $p > 0.05$].

The rest results are shown in Table 2.

Correlations between anxiety, depression and PTSD

The correlations between all variables were displayed in Table 1. There was a significantly positive correlation between anxiety and depression/ PTSD ($r = 0.594$, $p < 0.001$; $r = 0.517$, $p < 0.001$). The correlation between depression and PTSD was also significantly positive ($r = 0.469$, $p < 0.001$).

Discussion

Public health emergencies such as SARS and COVID-19 have sudden, public and serious social harmfulness (Main et al., 2011). During the Chinese Spring Festival, the outbreak of the COVID-19 has generated either direct or indirect impact on most parts of the society.

Our findings suggest that the prevalence of anxiety, depression and PTSD among the general public was 14.4, 29.7, and 5.6%, respectively during the period between January 26, 2020 and February 2, 2020, the two weeks into the country's outbreak of COVID-19, of which one week into the cities self-isolation policy. Also, at the same period WHO declared public health emergency of international concern.

Compared to the findings of a study focusing on the anxiety and depression among 3881 college students in Guangdong province under the context of COVID-19 pandemic, whose prevalence of anxiety and depression was 26.60 and 21.16%, respectively (Chang et al., 2020), the depression level in our study was high, while the anxiety level was relatively low. The inconsistency findings between the two studies may be due to the differences in the age structure of the participants. More than half of the participants in our study were college age students, but still 12 percent of the participants were over 45 years of age, and some were between 20 and 45 years old, and all of these participants had graduated from college. At the same time, some participants in our research were parents. Previous emergency related studies (Tan, 2003) have found that quite a lot of college students were lack of the experience to deal with public health emergencies. Their emotions are more suggestible, unstable and impulsive. In order to cope with the outbreak, colleges had delayed the start of school, and college students must go out less. As a result, college students were unable to carry out normal learning and social activities, which may affect their learning progress and aggravate their anxiety (Chang et al., 2020). Compared with college students who were self-isolating at home, essential workers had to go out. They had to wear masks when they went out, their temperature were taken many times when they were outside, and they had to disinfect them when they were back home. Some participants, like parents, carried more pressure as they needed to concern their families' health conditions.. In this case, older people may be more prone to depression than anxiety. This explained why the prevalence of this study was low in anxiety but high in depression comparing to the findings generated from pure college student samples..

The prevalence of invasion reached 47.8%, which was significantly higher than that of other dimensions of PTSD in our study. This may be related to the constant and repeating exposure of information about the epidemic from social media. In a study on the mental health and psychological state of college students during the COVID-19, the researchers found that the higher college students' awareness of COVID-19 was, the lower the likelihood of having mild anxiety (Chang et al., 2020). This indicated that the more comprehensive the understanding of COVID-19 among college students had, the better preventive measures they would have, and the more active they would be in dealing with the epidemic (Chang et al., 2020). Another study showed that during times of uncertainty and crisis, the public may increase their reliance on the media (Ball-Rokeach & DeFleur, 1976). These findings revealed that people tend to form accurate perceptions of risk when facts were known and been communicated to the public effectively via the media. During public health emergency, urgent messages must be delivered to the general public in real time, however, adverse media exposure that can lead to traumatic stress and related diseases must be reduced. A previous study (Garfin et al., 2020) showed that while the media must communicate information to the public to promote appropriate health protection behaviors and effective institutional responses, it must be communicated without sensational or disturbing images. In turn, the public should be recommended to avoid speculative stories, to limit repeated exposure to media stories with little new information, and to keep up with key updates. When misinformation is spread on social media, it may increase people's perception on risks and their fears of health-related topics (Wang et al., 2019), which makes the responsible use of social media imperative. Garfin's research (2020) also pointed that repeated media exposure to community crisis can lead to 1) increased anxiety, 2) heightened stress responses that can lead to downstream effects on health, and 3) misplaced health-protective and help-seeking behaviors that can overburden health care facilities and tax available resources. In other words, excessive media coverage of events generates unintended consequences for those at relatively low risk in direct exposure, leading to potentially severe public health repercussions. This may also help to explain the high prevalence of invasion in this study.

In our study, participants' scores on anxiety, depression and each dimension of PTSD showed high correlations, which is consistent with previous findings (Chang et al., 2020). In the following, we will discuss the significance of differences among groups in our findings. Participants under the age of 45 years old had higher scores in anxiety, depression and PTSD than those over the 45 years old; and the difference in anxiety between these two groups reached a significant level. Most of the young participants in our study were college or graduate students. In another study (Wang et al., 2020), students in schools were found to experience a psychological impact of the outbreak and reported higher levels of stress, anxiety, and depression compared to those who had graduated. As the total number of people infected by COVID-19 currently has surpasses that stricken by the 2003 SARS epidemic, major cities in China have shut down schools at all levels indefinitely. The uncertainty and potential negative impact on academic progression could have an adverse effect on the mental health of students. Young people also had more access to social media and social platforms, which increased their exposure to negative news under the epidemic. Mass repeated media exposure to community emergency can lead to increased anxiety and heightened stress responses ,and all of them can lead to health problems (Garfin et al., 2020).

Whether the participants' residency changed during the spring festival may also have an impact on their mental health and psychological state. The outbreak of the epidemic occurred around the Chinese Spring Festival, during which most of college students returned home as that's their winter vacation time, and migrant workers all over China also returned home to celebrate Spring Festival. Under the COVID-19, most Chinese people's' tourism plans had been canceled except going to their hometown to visit families. While massive population movements increased the risk of spreading the virus, returning to one's hometown to see relatives and families who had not been seen for a long time, still brought individual the sense of family connectivity. It may also play a certain role in the psychological health of individuals, and to some extent alleviate the degree of anxiety and depression under the epidemic. However, there was no significant difference in anxiety, depression, and PTSD levels between those who returned home and those who did not in our findings. This is contrary to our hypothesis. There were two possible explanations for this result. First, when returning home, individuals had to take the public transportation which typically are crowded. The crowdedness at public transportation increased risks in catching the virus under conditions of COVID-19 outbreak. People who had gone home before the information about COVID-19 was disclosed did not take any protective measures against COVID-19 when taking transportations. As a result, they may be infected and had the potential to pass on the danger to their families, which on the contrary increased their own and family menbers' anxiety and depression. Second, the scales in our study only measured individual levels of anxiety, depression, and PTSD, with very few questions involving families. Therefore, factors associated with family support may not be accurately detected by our survey. More information directly related to the family support is needed to acquire a more intuitive understanding of whether returning hometown can be a protective factors for an individual's mental state under the circumstance of COVID-19. As a result, whether returning hometown during the epidemic can relieve individual anxiety, depression, and PTSD levels still needs to be verified by future studies.

Implications

The results of the study shed light on the need to ensure mental health services in China when strict self-isolation policies are implemented in cities. We believe that the social media should report the situation of the epidemic fairly and convey important information to the public in time. We also suggest the relevant departments/sectors to strengthen the management of the self-media platform in order to let the audience avoid the repeated exposure of news or the excessive spread of rumors. People should know how to protect themselves by screening news in life, and receiving truly effective information. At the same time, we recommend people to keep doing things closely related to their daily life, through which to enhance the sense of control and the reality of life, in hope to cope with the inner sense of anxiety and loneliness caused by self-isolation.

Limitations

Our study adopts the snowball sampling strategy to enlarge the recruitment given the limitation in resources and the time sensitivity of COVID-19 outbreaks. This sampling strategy is not based on random selection of participants, nor does the study population reflect the actual distribution of the general population. In addition, if we can follow up the same group of participants after a period of time to observe the changes of their mental health and psychological state over time, it will certainly provide us with more information. However, due to the ethical requirements of anonymity and confidentiality, we could not collect contact information and personal information from participants. Therefore, there is no way to obtain long-term data. Another limitation is that self-reported levels of anxiety, depression, and PTSD may not always be consistent with the assessment done by mental health professionals. Similarly, respondents, even when completing anonymous questionnaires, may have provided responses to meet the social expectations when reporting psychological states, without reporting their real states. There was an oversampling of a particular network of similar groups (e.g., college students), leading to selection bias. As a result, the conclusion was less generalizable to the entire population, particularly less educated people and children.

Conclusion

It is thus concluded that COVID-19 had adverse effects on the self-isolating populations, causing severe symptoms of anxiety, depression and PTSD to them. Compare to pure college student group, we found that complex group may having more severe mental health problems like depression due to the outbreak of COVID-19. The distribution difference of outcome variables in demographic variables demonstrated that younger people were more likely to develop the symptoms of anxiety, depression and PTSD than the older people when facing this kind of public health emergencies, such as COVID-19. Besides, because of high contagiousness, people all around the country (northern, southwest and eastern of China) are equally vulnerable to get impacted directly or indirectly. What's more, the excessive media exposure may lead to PTSD through over invasion. Given the potentially negative impact of COVID-19 on self-isolating population's mental health, efforts are needed in the directions mentioned above to enhance the mental health support services for the self-isolating general public.

Acknowledgments

We extend our gratitude to the researchers in the psychology field who volunteered to help us spread the questionnaire around. We also appreciate the participants for their time and efforts in completing our surveys while coping with COVID-19.

Disclosure statement

The author(s) declared no potential conflict of interest with respect to this research, authorship, and/or the publication of this article.

Author contributions

All authors contributed to the study conception and design. The first draft of the manuscript was written by [Yu qing Zhao] and all authors commented on previous versions of the manuscript. All authors read and approved the final manuscript.

Funding

This research was supported by The National Science Foundation of the Jiangsu Higher Education Institutions of China [Project No. 18KJB190004] and The Philosophy and Social Science Foundation of Jiangsu [Project No. 18SHC004] and Philosophy and The Social Sciences of Jiangsu Higher Education Institutions [Project No. 2018SJZDI206].

References

American Psychiatric Association. (2013). *Diagnostic and statistical manual of mental disorders (DSM-5®)*. American Psychiatric Pub.

An, Y., Huang, J., Chen, Y., & Deng, Z. (2019, March 25). *Longitudinal Cross-Lagged Relationships Between Posttraumatic Stress Disorder and Depression in Adolescents Following the Yancheng Tornado in China. Psychological Trauma: Theory, Research, Practice, and Policy*. Advance online publication. http://dx.doi.org/10.1037/tra0000455

Ball-Rokeach, S. J., & DeFleur, M. L. (1976). A dependency model of mass-media effects. *Communication Research*, *3*(1), 3–21. http://dx.doi.org/10.1177/009365027600300101.

Blevins, C. A., Weathers, F. W., Davis, M. T., Witte, T. K., & Domino, J. L. (2015). The Posttraumatic Stress Disorder Checklist for DSM-5 (PCL-5): Development and Initial Psychometric Evaluation. *Journal of Traumatic Stress*, *28*(6), 489–498. https://doi.org/10.1002/jts.22059

CCTV News (2020, January 26). Has the virus mutated? Will there be more cities locken down? Will the vacation be extended? The national health commission responded one by one. https://mp.weixin.qq.com/s/W8rQ8T46qV0pxHs03sF6hw.

Chang, J., Yuan, Y., & Wang, D. (2020). Mental health status and its influencing factors among college students during the epidemic of COVID-19. *Journal of South Medicine University*, *40*(2), 171–176. https://doi.org/10.12122/j.issn.1673-4254.2020.02.06.

Cui, J., Li, F., & Shi, Z. L. (2019). Origin and evolution of pathogenic coronaviruses. *Nature Reviews Microbiology*, *17*(3), 181–192. https://doi.org/10.1038/s41579-018-0118-9.

Garfin, D. R., Silver, R. C., & Holman, E. A. (2020, March 23). The novel coronavirus (COVID-2019) outbreak: Amplification of public health consequences by media exposure. *Health Psychology*, *39*(5), 355–357. http://dx.doi.org/10.1037/hea0000875.

Giummarra, M. J., Lennox, A., Dali, G., Costa, B., & Gabbe, B. J. (2018, August 2017). Early psychological interventions for posttraumatic stress, depression and anxiety after traumatic injury: A systematic review and meta-analysis. *Clinical Psychology Review*, *62*, 11–36. https://doi.org/10.1016/j.cpr.2018.05.001

Khazaie, H., Ghadami, M. R., & Masoudi, M. (2016). Sleep disturbances in veterans with chronic war-induced PTSD. *Journal of Injury & Violence Research*, *8*(2), 99–107. https://doi.org/10.5249/jivr.v8i2.808

Li, J., Wang, S., Yu, R., Hu, J., Jiang, M., & Huang, W. (2020). Compliance of home quarantine protection and its effext on anxiety degree during the epidemic outbreak period of COVID-19. *Journal Chinese Control Infection*, *19*(4), 1–7.

Liu, K., Chen, Y., Wu, D., Lin, R., Wang, Z., & Pan, L. (2020). Effects of progressive muscle relaxation on anxiety and sleep quality in patients with COVID-19. *Complementary Therapies in Clinical Practice*, *39*, 101132. https://doi.org/10.1016/j.ctcp.2020.101132.

Liu, N., Zhang, F., Wei, C., Jia, Y., Shang, Z., Sun, L., Wu, L., Sun, Z., Zhou, Y., Wang, Y., & Liu, W. (2020). Prevalence and predictors of PTSS during COVID-19 outbreak in China hardest-hit areas: Gender differences matter. *Psychiatry Research*, *287*, 112921. https://doi.org/10.1016/j.psychres.2020.112921

Mahmoud, J. S. R., Staten, R. T., Hall, L. A., & Lennie, T. A. (2012). The relationship among young adult college students' depression, anxiety, stress, demographics, life satisfaction, and coping styles. *Issues in Mental Health Nursing*, *33*(3), 149–156. https://doi.org/10.3109/01612840.2011.632708.

Main, A., Zhou, Q., Ma, Y., Luecken, L. J., & Liu, X. (2011). Relations of SARS-related stressors and coping to Chinese college students' psychological adjustment during the

2003 Beijing SARS epidemic. *Journal of Counseling Psychology, 58*(3), 410–423. https://doi.org/10.1037/a0023632

Podsakoff, P. M., Mackenzie, S. B., Lee, J.-Y., & Podsakoff, N. P. (2003). Common method biases in behavioral research: A critical review of the literature and recommended remedies. *Journal of Applied Psychology, 88*(5), 879–903. https://doi.org/10.1037/0021-9010.88.5.879

Qiu, J., Shen, B., Zhao, M., Wang, Z., Xie, B., & Xu, Y. (2020). A nationwide survey of psychological distress among Chinese people in the COVID-19: implications and policy recommendations. *General Psychiatry, 33*(2), e100213–21. https://doi.org/10.1136/gpsych-2020-100213.

Rajkumar, R. P. (2020). COVID-19 and mental health: a review of the existing literature. *Asian Journal of Psychiatry, 52,* 102066. https://doi.org/https://doi.org/10.1016/j.ajp.2020.102066.

Slovic, P., & Peters, E. (2006). Risk perception and affect. *Current Directions in Psychological Science, 15*(6), 322–325. https://doi.org/10.1111/j.1467-8721.2006.00461.x.

Tan, X. D. (2003). *Prevention and control of sudden public health events [M]* (p. 45). Hubei Health Publishing House.

Wang, Y., McKee, M., Torbica, A., & Stuckler, D. (2019). Systematic literature review on the spread of health-related misinformation on social media. *Social Science & Medicine, 240,* 112552. http://dx.doi.org/10.1016/j.socscimed.2019.112552.

Wang, C., Pan, R., Wan, X., Tan, Y., Xu, L., Ho, C. S., & Ho, R. C. (2020). Immediate psychological responses and associated factors during the initial stage of the 2019 coronavirus disease (COVID-19) epidemic among the general population in China. *International Journal of Environmental Research and Public Health, 17*(5), 1729. https://doi.org/10.3390/ijerph17051729.

World Health Organization (2020, January 30). Statement on the second meeting of the International Health Regulations(2005)Emergency Committee regarding the outbreak of novel coronavirus(2019-nCoV). https://www.who.int/news-room/detail/30-01-2020-statement-on-the-second-meeting-of-the-international-health-regulations-(2005)-emergency-committee-regarding-the-outbreak-of-novel-coronavirus-(2019-ncov).

Zhong, B. L., Ruan, Y. F., Xu, Y. M., Chen, W. C., & Liu, L. F. (2020, September 2019). Prevalence and recognition of depressive disorders among Chinese older adults receiving primary care: A multi-center cross-sectional study. *Journal of Affective Disorders, 260,* 26–31. https://doi.org/10.1016/j.jad.2019.09.011.

Zung, W. W. (1971). A rating instrument for anxiety disorders. *Psychosomatics, 12*(6), 371–379. https://doi.org/10.1016/S0033-3182(71)71479-0.

Zung, W. W., Richards, C. B., & Short, M. J. (1965). Self-Rating Depression Scale in an outpatient clinic: Further validation of the SDS. *Archives of General Psychiatry, 13*(6), 508–515. https://doi.org/10.1001/archpsyc.1965.01730060026004.

A Glimpse of University Students' Family Life Amidst the COVID-19 Virus

Haimin Pan

ABSTRACT
This essay uses a small-scale set of data derived from university students whom I can contact during this period. The variables were particularly pertinent to their family life amidst the COVID-19 virus, including, but not limited to, learning experience with online courses, evaluation on the Government measures against the COVID-19 virus spread, perception of the influence of the pestilence on their own thoughts and behaviors. A simple calculation of frequency was adopted to present the situation related. Results showed a unique experience of the students in the situation of the COVID-19 virus, and reflection on those results was available.

It has been nearly one month since I came to Xiamen City Fujian Province of China for transfer of work on 29 February 2020 from Wenzhou City where the spread of the COVID-19 virus is relatively concerning as compared to other cities exclusive of many cities in Hubei province. I first took medical quarantine for 14 days at a hotel and afterward lived as usual with freedom walking around. I thought of this kind of measure as necessary and effective, as well as other ones (e.g., wearing facemasks, regular hand hygiene, and staying at home). And washing hands regularly may be more important than facemask use in preventing influenza transmission (Saunders-Hastings et al., 2017). Everyone's lifestyle has changed since the existence of COVID-19 virus. I did an online survey among my students these two days reflecting their family life as they were now staying at home and taking part in online courses. Twenty questions were designed to have a glimpse of their family life amidst the COVID-19 virus, including, but not limited to, learning experience with online courses, evaluation of the Government measures against the COVID-19 virus spread, perception of the influence of the pestilence on their own thoughts and behaviors. Ninety-four students filled in this online survey and provided answers to the questions related. They came from Gansu, Zhejiang, Fujian,

Guangdong, and other 16 provinces in mainland China. The following paragraphs center on the results of this survey.

In terms of the students' learning experience of online courses, mobile telephone (93.85%) and laptop (75.38%) were the two types of electronic equipment that were used by the majority of them for accessing the online course, apart from the pad (16.92%) and desk computer (13.85%). 81.91% of the students regarded online courses as necessary before they were allowed for returning to the campus. As for the online course, live telecast, rather than recorded broadcast, of the courses was the first choice of the majority of the students (76.60%). Nearly half of the students took the online courses with a length of 30–60 minutes (46.15%), followed by 91–120 minutes (21.54%) and 61–90 minutes (16.92%). Among them, a course delivered online within 30–60 minutes was most fond of by the students (72.34%), followed by others, for example, of 61–90 minutes (14.89%) and of less than 30 minutes (7.45%).

Regarding the students' activities in their spare time, watching TV (73.4%), reading books (68.09%), writing papers (64.89%), and playing computer games (56.38%) were frequently engaged by the students. The degree of care of the students about the severity situation of COVID-19 virus varied. Exactly 38.30% of the students searched for news about the epidemic per day, and 26.6% of them did so usually. And part of them sometimes (24.47%) or occasionally (10.64%) initiatively searched for news about the epidemic situation. Overall, some students (39.36%) felt somewhat boring dating at home, and 26.60% of them perceived family life during the special time as so-so and 15.96% not boring. Whereas, 10.64 and 7.45% of the students felt extremely boring or extremely enriched.

Although personal hygiene was highly emphasized, there was a small proportion of the students (14.89%) who thought that they did not pay more attention to personal hygiene than before. To be noted, 75.53% of the students deemed that wearing facemasks when going outside would be compulsory and beneficial for themselves even when the epidemic is under control and vanishes. The importance attached to the facemasks use was consistent with how the student felt about the COVID-19 virus transmission. In this sense, 82.98% of the students were fearful of this emergent public health event and 52.13% of them chose not to go to Hubei provinces or other cities where the epidemic was serious.

In general, most of the students (91.49%) positively evaluated the effectiveness of the measures and interventions taken by the central and/or local governments. Regarding their own contribution to this public health event, 84.04% of the student perceived themselves to be contributive, say, in the aspects of personal hygiene, donation, and being volunteers. Some students also pointed out that staying at home was contributory. Only 15.96% of the students perceived that they did not contribute to this big event.

The results showed a different learning experience in the situation of COVID-19 virus from the time when they were on campus before. Gradually they get used to taking courses via the Internet. Particularly, activities unique to the COVID-19 virus spread include donation, personal hygiene, their preference for traveling to the cities ever in major transmission, and their feeling about this public health event. It can be seen that the large-scale transmission renders the students become careful about their personal health and conscious about what they can do for society. Noted, many students perceived staying at home is a form of a contribution to controlling the COVID-19 virus transmission apart from other behaviors, like donation and being volunteers. Yang et al. (2006) revealed that common people got anxious during the SARS crisis. According to the statement of the students, it is the same case this time as 82.98% of the students felt fearful of this emergent public health event. Similarly, a recent study showed that people's negative emotions and sensitivity to social risk have increased since the official declaration of COVID-19 (Li et al., 2020). According to the previous findings, it is believed that the effective preventive actions of government and recovery information in effect could ameliorate people's risk perception of their self-interests and their families (Shi et al., 2003). It is inferred that the role of the government is of utmost importance. This accord with the social administration pattern in China. Nowadays, the influence of COVID-19 virus has become worldwide, and as compared to other countries, China has attained the lowest scores in terms of the insufficient reactions from the government, but achieved a relatively high level of trust from its citizens (Roth et al., 2020).

Overall, this emergent public health event is influencing everyone's life. The glimpse of university students' family life amidst the COVID-19 virus reflects the reactions and perceptions of them in a special period. I hope the spring will come soon and smile blossoms in people's faces after the outbreak.

References

Li, S., Wang, Y., Xue, J., Zhao, N., & Zhu, T. (2020). The impact of COVID 19 epidemic declaration on psychological consequences: A study on active Weibo users. *International Journal of Environmental Research and Public Health, 17*(6), 2032. doi:10.3390/ijerph17062032

Roth, C., Caria, S., Fetzer, T., Hensel, L., Gómez, M., Haushofer, J., & Goetz, F. (2020). *Measuring worldwide COVID-19 attitudes and beliefs*. International Survey on Coronavirus. http://www.covid19-survey.org

Saunders-Hastings, P., Crispo, J. A. G., Sikora, L., & Krewski, D. (2017). Effectiveness of personal protective measures in reducing pandemic influenza transmission: A systematic review and meta-analysis. *Epidemics*, *20*, 1–20. doi:10.1016/j.epidem.2017.04.003

Shi, K., Fan, H., Jia, J., Li, W., Song, Z., Gao, J., & Hu, W. (2003). The risk perceptions of SARS and socio-psychological behaviors of urban people in China. *Acta Psychologica Sinica*, *35*(4), 546–554.

Yang, C., Wang, Y., Pan, J., & Wen, S. (2006). The impact of the SARS on the mentality and behaviors of the different population (in Chinese). *Journal of Tropical Medicine*, *6*(2), 159–161.

Stranded College Students amid Corona Virus Disease 2019 Pandemic: An Existential Phenomenology

Michael B. Cahapay

ABSTRACT
This paper explores the lived experiences of college students who are stranded in the middle of the Corona Virus Disease 2019 (COVID-19) crisis. It follows the approach of Heideggerian existential phenomenology in studying ontology or what it means to be. Five college students were purposively selected to participate in the study. The researcher gained insight into each world of the students using interview procedures and thematic analysis. The results are presented through emerging themes and contextual ground. A conceptual structure that depicts the essence of the lived experiences of the stranded college students is offered in the end of the paper.

Introduction

Since the public announcement about it (Li et al., 2020) and eventual outbreak from Wuhan, China (Phelan et al., 2020), the COVID-19 has created an unprecedented crisis in the world. The education sector is neither spared as students are considered as one of the most vulnerable groups. The International Association of Universities (2020), an independent global organization affiliated with UNESCO, initially reported that more than a billion and a half students across the world are affected by school closures due to the COVID-19 outbreak.

In the Philippine educational setting, stranded college students are a major concern. The Commission on Higher Education responded by assisting these college students stranded within and outside the country to go back to their hometowns (Bernardo, 2020). Save the Children Philippines (2020), a private organization reported a call for schools to prevent the effects of class disruptions caused by the COVID-19 quarantine. However, despite the efforts to help stranded students, Wong (2020) wrote about the inevitable impacts of the ensuing COVID-19.

As far as the most recent pandemics such as the H1N1 and the current COVID-19 are concerned, review of empirical studies about lived experiences using phenomenology as a research approach mostly focused on allied medical fields as well as school job context (e.g. Corley et al., 2010; Guillaume et al., 2019; Howard & Howard, 2012; Raymond et al., 2019; Van et al., 2010; Wang et al., 2020). However, of equal interest, is the need to account for the lived experiences of a vulnerable group of stranded students who are at risk of psychosocial pressures.

A description of the lived experiences of college students who are stranded due to pandemic is significant in the current theory, practice, and research. Thus, the purpose of this paper is to explore the lived experiences of stranded college students amid the COVID-19 crisis.

Methods

An existential phenomenology is entailed in this research. It is found appropriate because it focuses more on ontology or what it means to be (Heidegger, 1962/1999) in the context of the COVID-19 pandemic. The participants were five college students from a university in Mindanao, Philippines. They were not able to return to their respective homes and are stranded since the declaration of the community quarantine. The researcher sought to gain insight into each world of stranded students through the use of interview procedures and thematic analysis. An augmented form called online interview was done. It is an accepted research method conducted using communication mediated by computers (Salmons, 2014). The researcher further interpreted the lived experiences of the stranded students through thematic analysis. The theme is the main product of this analysis technique (Green et al., 2007).

Results

Emerging themes

The construct and concepts generated from the master transcript of the responses of the participants resulted in the identification of emerging themes of the lived experiences of the stranded college students. They are described as follows.

Theme 1: Riding through an "emotional rollercoaster"

There appeared to be no single emotion, but an "emotional rollercoaster" of different reactions (Amundson & Borgen, 1987) as the participants experienced the COVID-19 pandemic in the different stages.

First, before the pandemic, the participants recalled that they seemed not to mind the initial crisis as they were busy complying requirements in school ("During that time my hands were full of school requirements, so I did not mind." – Kristine). This oblivious emotion persisted even up to the first week of class suspension when the initial positive COVID-19 cases in the country were reported. However, as the class suspension was extended and the number of positive COVID-19 cases surged, the participants began to feel a sense of alarm culminating in a shock when community quarantine was placed, severely restricting movement ("It was getting alarming as the suspension prolonged and I became worried" – Carlos). This pandemic stage produced expressions of concerns. The participants conveyed anxiety about unfinished school requirements, scarce food supplies, and uncertain family situations. Finally, in the present pandemic stage, the participants experienced mixed emotions of loneliness, regret, and frustration ("I was so sad and frustrated. I wanted to go home but I could not" – Juana).

Theme 2: Embracing a "new normal"

During the COVID-19 situation, new habits and practices which were previously considered not normal have become normal. The participants observed "new normal" (El-Erian, 2010) as they lived day to day in the last two months.

The participants noticed that some changes in their routines, both positive and negative, have taken place ("I do some stuff I don't usually do, like cooking my food, sleep as much as I can, and have a lot of idle time" – Carlos). They found a way to cope with their studies ("During this COVID-19 crisis I developed an easier method to memorize some terms." – Liam). They also observed the cultivation of their leisure skills to a greater degree ("I was able to develop my cooking skills and was able to perfect some of my recipes" – Juana). New lifestyles had also to be adopted ("Extending the food supply I have for a week into a month" – Andrew).

Theme 3: Undergoing a "growth under pressure"

The participants further described their experiences through the use of positive approaches to overcome the impacts brought by the COVID-19 predicament. These approaches can be summed up to the expression "growth under pressure" (Monteiro, 1990) as the participants gained positive insights from the situation.

The situation turned the participants to become more vigilant and take their responsibilities as citizens ("When the authority mandates to stay at home, it is our role to follow it" – Kristine). They practiced proactive means to regulate their emotions ("Being calm is the best way to make ourselves safe." – Liam). They also realized that some of the most essential things in life are immaterial ("It made me realize that money has no value in times like this" - Andrew). Other participants cited the value of their families in the distance in crisis ("We should never take our families for granted and that families should always come first" - Juana).

Contextual ground

The analysis of the lived experiences of the stranded college students needed to be understood in a context. It showed that the context of the participants is grounded against space from which their experiences emerge. This concept of space was drawn from one of the four existential worlds that guide reflections on the phenomenon (Dowling, 2007).

First, the "real space" is the space from which the participants physically exist. During the public emergency caused by COVID-19, the participants as stranded college students described their real space as a space where they express their response to the phenomenon. They expressed that:

> "Going out is strictly prohibited nowadays and my actions are limited. I just do my everyday routine which makes me feel less productive" (Carlos).
>
> "Surviving with the little food that I have, I planted some vegetables from the knowledge I learned from school. From then on, I was able to survive" (Andrew).

Moreover, the existence of a "wished space" is reified in the narratives of the experiences of the participants as stranded college students. It is the space that they desire to exist but could not because of the pandemic that restricted their movement. They vented out that:

> "It has been about two months since the last time that I went home and every single day that I'm away makes me ask myself: When will I be home?" (Juana).
>
> "It is not easy because you are far apart from your hometown and you don't know if you can still come home or not" (Liam).

Lastly, there is also a "virtual space." The role of "virtual space" as a bridge between the "real space" and "wished space" is manifested by the reactions of the participants as they struggle with the restriction brought by the pandemic. They stated that:

> "Since I can barely go outside, I use social media and other applications which are relatively useful for better communication to my relatives and friends" (Carlos).
>
> "I think online messaging applications helped a lot. I and my family can exchange video calls almost every day, so it helped ease the homesickness" (Juana).

Conceptual structure

The interrelationships found among the three themes and the three spaces illustrate the conceptual structure of the lived experiences of the stranded college students (Figure 1).

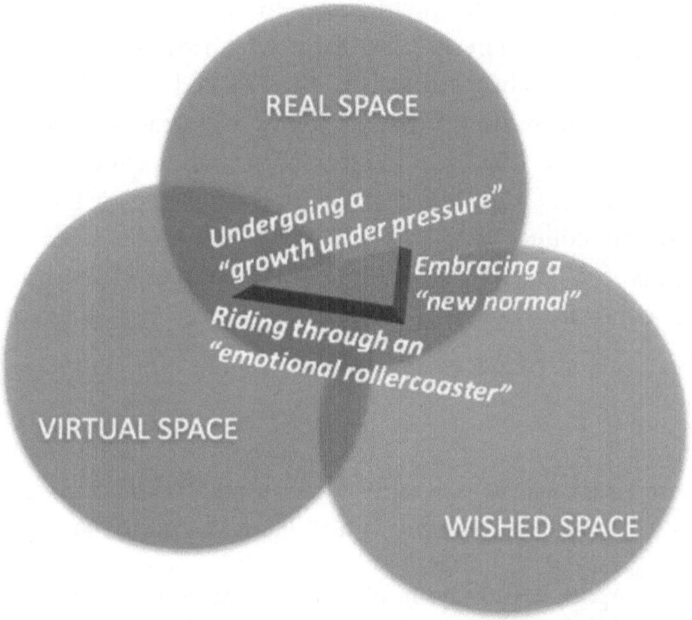

Figure 1. Conceptual structure of lived experiences of stranded college students.

The emerging themes are placed in the shape of an upended triangle, implying an interconnection that is not necessarily hierarchical but contributory ("I was thinking of what to eat for the next days or months [emotional rollercoaster] ... Extending the food supply I have for a week into a month [new normal] ... I planted some vegetables from the knowledge I learned from school [growth under pressure]" – Andrew). The theme located above the triangle denotes a positive message of resolution of the two other themes below. The three themes are within the overlapping portion of the contextual ground, which means that each stands out from the integrated nature of the three spaces.

The contextual ground is represented by three circles for the "real space," "wished space," and "virtual space." The circles are overlapping, denoting that each space is interconnected. This nature of the circles denotes that the participants struggle as they experience each fully ("I wanted to go home [wished space] ... but ... I had a lot of unfinished things at school [real space]. I think online messaging applications helped [virtual space] ... " – Juana). The positions and colors of the circles represent the relative prominence of each world to the participant. The real space is placed at the top while the wished space is located at the bottom.

Conclusion

Three themes represent the essence of the lived experiences of stranded college students. These themes highlight the experiences of riding through an "emotional rollercoaster," embracing a "new normal," and undergoing a "growth under pressure." The ground from which these themes are situated consists of three spaces: the "real space," the "wished space," and the "virtual space." The relationships among these themes and spaces illustrate the conceptual structure of the lived experiences of stranded college students. This paper presents evidence that leads to an understanding of the lived experiences of stranded college students. By exploring these lived experiences, it offers inputs for the development of various mechanisms that will improve the conditions of this vulnerable group in times of unprecedented crisis.

References

Amundson, N. E., & Borgen, W. A. (1987). The dynamics of unemployment. *Journal of Counseling & Development, 66*(4), 180–184. https://doi.org/10.1002/j.1556-6676.1987.tb00841.x

Bernardo, J. (2020, April). CHED says helping stranded students get home amid COVID-19 travel restrictions. *ABS-CBN News*. https://news.abs-cbn.com/news/04/29/20/ched-says-helping-stranded-students-get-home-amid-covid-19-travel-restrictions

Corley, A., Hammond, N. E., & Fraser, J. F. (2010). The experiences of health care workers employed in an Australian intensive care unit during the H1N1 Influenza pandemic of 2009: A phenomenological study. *International Journal of Nursing Studies, 47*(5), 577–585. https://doi.org/10.1016/j.ijnurstu.2009.11.015

Dowling, M. (2007). From Husserl to van Manen. A review of different phenomenological approaches. *International Journal of Nursing Studies, 44*(1), 131–142. https://doi.org/10.1016/j.ijnurstu.2005.11.026.

El-Erian, M. A. (2010). *Navigating the new normal in industrial countries*. International Monetary Fund.

Green, J., Willis, K., Hughes, E., Small, R., Welch, N., Gibbs, L., & Daly, J. (2007). Generating best evidence from qualitative research: The role of data analysis. *Australian and New Zealand Journal of Public Health, 31*(6), 545–550. https://doi.org/10.1111/j.1753-6405.2007.00141.x

Guillaume, Y., Raymond, M., Jerome, G. J., Ternier, R., & Ivers, L. C. (2019). 'It was a ravage!': lived experiences of epidemic cholera in rural Haiti. *BMJ Global Health, 4*(6), e001834. https://doi.org/10.1136/bmjgh-2019-001834

Heidegger, M. (1962/1999). Exposition of the question of the meaning of being. In C. Polifroni & M. Welch (Eds.), *Perspectives on philosophy of science in nursing* (pp. 273–301). Lippincott.

Howard, P., & Howard, J. (2012). Pandemic and pedagogy: Elementary school teachers' experience of H1N1 Influenza in the classroom. *Phenomenology & Practice*, *6*(1), 18–35. https://doi.org/10.29173/pandpr19852.

International Association of Universities. (2020, April 25). *COVID-19: Higher education challenges and responses* [Report]. https://www.iau-aiu.net/Covid-19-Higher-Education-challenges-and-responses

Li, Q., Guan, X., Wu, P., Wang, X., Zhou, L., Tong, Y., Ren, R., Leung, K. S. M., Lau, E. H. Y., Wong, J. Y., Xing, X., Xiang, N., Wu, Y., Li, C., Chen, Q., Li, D., Liu, T., Zhao, J., Liu, M., … Feng, Z. (2020). Early transmission dynamics in Wuhan, China, of novel coronavirus-infected pneumonia. *The New England Journal of Medicine*, *382*(13), 1199–1069. https://doi.org/10.1056/NEJMoa2001316

Monteiro, G. (1990). Hemingway's notion of "grace. *Studies in American Fiction*, *18*(1), 111–112. https://doi.org/10.1353/saf.1990.0025.

Phelan, A. L., Katz, R., & Gostin, L. O. (2020). The novel coronavirus originating in Wuhan, China: challenges for global health governance. *JAMA*, *323*(8), 709–710. https://doi.org/10.1001/jama.2020.1097

Salmons, J. (2014). *Qualitative online interviews: Strategies, design, and skills.* Sage Publications, Inc.

Save the Children Philippines. (2020, March 12). *Children not spared from the impacts of the virus on society as a global pandemic is declared, warns Save the Children Philippines* [Story]. https://www.savethechildren.org.ph/our-work/our-stories/story/covid-19/

Van, D., McLaws, M. L., Crimmins, J., MacIntyre, C. R., & Seale, H. (2010). University life and pandemic influenza: Attitudes and intended behaviour of staff and students towards pandemic (H1N1). *BMC Public Health*, *10*(1), 130. https://doi.org/10.1186/1471-2458-10-130.

Wang, N., Duan, W., He, X., Li, X. (2020). *Lived experience of individuals fighting against the panic and discrimination under the COVID-19 pandemic in China.* https://www.iassw-aiets.org

Wong, B. (2020, March). Universities are failing their students during the coronavirus outbreak. *Times Higher Education.* https://www.timeshighereducation.com/blog/universities-are-failing-their-students-during-coronavirus-outbreak.

A Researcher and Survivor of the Holocaust Connect and Make Meaning during the COVID-19 Pandemic

Carolyn Ellis and Jerry Rawicki

ABSTRACT
This article features an interview conducted on April 20th, 2020 with Jerry Rawicki, a 93-year-old survivor of the Holocaust, about his experience during the COVID-19 Pandemic and how it compares to what happened to him during the Holocaust. The first author reflects briefly on her own experience of the pandemic and how she decided to focus on Jerry's story. The frustrations and successes in using social media technology to conduct interviews are described. The article concludes with a discussion of connecting and engaging in meaningful activity as two significant ways to cope with our anxieties, fears, and sense of isolation during the pandemic.

"What about the pandemic bothers you the most?" I ask Jerry.

"The unknown. I don't know what's going to happen and not knowing makes me imagine all kinds of things. I am seeing in my mind's eye scenes of the Holocaust when we did without food and necessities. I know I shouldn't be comparing the two because the privation and the problems now and those that we had during the Holocaust are diametrically different. But who knows. This situation we're in might all change for the worst. That's what I'm worried about."

***

This article features an interview I (Carolyn), a writer and a scholar, conducted with Jerry Rawicki, a 93-year-old survivor of the Holocaust, about his experience during the COVID-19 pandemic and how it compares to what happened to him during the Holocaust. I first reflect briefly on my own experience of the pandemic and how I moved from my life to focus on Jerry's story. Then I discuss the frustrations and successes of using unfamiliar social media technology to do research when participants are separated by sheltering-in-place mandates. We conclude with a discussion of connecting and engaging in meaningful activity as two significant ways to cope with our anxieties, fears, and sense of isolation during the pandemic.

Deciding which story to tell

For the last thirty-five years, I (Carolyn) have written personal stories as a way to help me understand and live through trauma and chaos. For example, I wrote about my brother's death in a commercial airplane crash (Ellis, 1993), taking care of my mother who was ill (Ellis, 1996), the illness and death of my partner (1995/2018), and my experiences during the September 11, 2001 attacks on the World Trade Center (Ellis, 2002). In each of these cases, writing helped when little else offered any relief. But now I feel stymied. The COVID-19 Pandemic seems massive, overwhelming, and unpredictable as each day the deaths go up and we wait for the curve to flatten. What if it doesn't? What if it does and then rises again? What if a safe vaccine can't be developed?

The forecasts on COVID-19 from the experts at the University of Washington, statistics from Worldometer, and briefings and advice from government officials change daily. What is unthinkable one day becomes thinkable the next. What feels like an unbearable story one minute is superseded by something more horrible the next: frontline workers reusing N-95 masks, emergency personnel without sufficient PPE, doctors deciding who gets the last ICU bed and who should be connected to the last ventilator, essentially who should live and who could die. My experience seems insignificant compared to these stories and others that dominate the nightly news about workers losing jobs with no means of support; parents trying to work at home, take care of children, and provide homeschool simultaneously; entire families getting sick with the virus; workers on the front line experiencing symptoms; hospital workers facing unimaginable trauma in emergency rooms; and people dying alone while their families grieve in isolation, unable to see or attend a funeral service for their loved one. So many powerful stories circulate through the media.[1]

Still, I wake each day feeling the pull to write something that might help me and others to understand our experience of sheltering in place while feeling fear and facing unpredictability of what our lives have and may become. While THE story of COVID-19 evolves and changes every day—how many die or might die; the importance of sheltering in place vs. opening up the economy; the comparison of the virus to the common flu or to the Flu Pandemic of 1918; the mandate to wear a mask or not to wear a mask—by the middle of April, my story has taken on a day-to-day sameness. Mine is thankfully a boring tale about an advantaged life, where our long-term cook delivers healthy meals once a week to my partner Art and me. I am connected to my friends and family around the globe through text, email, phone, skype, and zoom.

In reality, my life has not been shattered by the virus though, as with others, it has been severely disrupted. As Peggy Noonan (2020) writes (with attribution to a tweet by Damian Barr), "We are not all in the same boat. We are all in the same storm. Some are in yachts and some have just the one oar." I may not be sheltering in a yacht, but I am fortunate to have both oars, and a spare one on hand should I need it. Retired and not teaching, I don't have chaos stories to tell of trying to teach online or assist students who are homeless or unable to connect on the internet. I don't have children who need care and consoling. While I miss going out and seeing people, I have resources, money still in my substantial but shrinking 401(k), a beautiful home with a fenced in backyard, a second home in the mountains in case we want to escape Florida, a partner with whom I enjoy sheltering in place and share intimacy, an old familiar dog of sixteen years to cuddle, and a new puppy to keep us entertained. I check in on friends and family, but I have minimal responsibilities at this stage of my life.

Do readers want to hear about my COVID-19 conversation with a neighbor I rarely talk to? The experience of watching the "Handmaid's Tale" in the middle of the pandemic? How the nightly news punctuates my and Art's moods and plays into our relationship? My continuing exercise program? My grief over our dog Zen who died just days before we began to take the virus seriously? The graceful aging of our ancient rat terrier who almost died after her canine companion passed and now has renewed life spurred on by our new puppy? Or the energy it takes to train five-month-old Malee, rewarded by watching her antics, and receiving her kisses and snuggles while many living alone have nobody to hug and touch? These all are stories in their own right and I have begun writing several of them. But I think they are stories for another time and another context when (or if) COVID-19 ceases dominating our concerns and we have space and energy to dwell again on living daily lives, coping with loss that happens for reasons other than the virus, and connecting to our canine companions.

The question I confront now is: do I want to glue myself to my computer to write about grief and loss, as I've done most of my life, especially during traumatic moments? What if the world as we know it really is ending? Or at least changing drastically in ways that are still unknowable and unthinkable? Is spending this time recording my experience better than soaking up experience, meditating and reflecting, connecting with others, or dedicating myself to helping those in need, or even reading a good novel?

Among my weekly check-ins is my friend and research partner Jerry, a survivor of the Holocaust. Jerry was twelve years old when Germany invaded Poland and he was deported from his native city of Plock to the small town of Bodzentyn. Together with his older sister, he made his way to the Warsaw Ghetto, where he became a courier between the budding Jewish resistance and the Polish underground. In April of 1943, he fought in the Warsaw Ghetto uprising, living for some time among rats in a burned out cellar where he subsisted on rotten potatoes. He escaped its smoldering ruins weeks after the Ghetto had fallen by climbing through a hole in the Ghetto wall. His mother and younger sister were gassed at Treblinka, his father died in a work camp, and his older sister survived by passing as Gentile in Warsaw. With the help of forged identification provided by the Polish underground, Jerry survived the remainder of the war by passing as a Roman Catholic. At the age of twenty-one, he arrived in New York in 1949, where he became an optician, and then later retired to Florida.

I have been working with Jerry for close to a dozen years. We have written about his experience during the Holocaust (Ellis & Rawicki, 2019; Rawicki & Ellis, 2011), the methodological approaches of compassionate interviewing and collaborative witnessing (Ellis & Rawicki, 2013; see also Ellis & Patti, 2014), and our mutual disrespect for Donald Trump and his similarity to Hitler (Ellis & Rawicki, 2018). Jerry lives with his daughter in St. Petersburg, 40 miles from me and we visit frequently. But due to COVID-19 I have not seen him now for several months and I miss our time together. In addition to not wanting to violate the shelter-in-place mandates and risk my and my partner Art's lives, I am doubly concerned about protecting Jerry who has lung and heart conditions in addition to being 93 years old.

As Jerry and I talk, I begin to realize that much might be learned by focusing on how a person who survived the Holocaust is experiencing this pandemic that has swept across the world. How do Jerry's experiences *then* play into what he is going through *now*? How do these two situations compare? What thoughts, feelings, and memories are provoked by the depiction of COVID-19 victims and survivors? How do survivors experience trauma, grief, and loss in their later years (Ellis & Patti, 2014)?

"Jerry," I say, interrupting our usual chat about Trump's latest antics.

"Yes?"

"How would you like to be interviewed about the pandemic?"

"I'd love it, but what do I have to offer?" I tell him why I think his particular experience is worth exploring. "I'm game. How do we proceed?"

Thus begins a conversation between two senior citizens, Jerry at 93 and me at 69, about COVID-19. Before moving to the content of our interview, I describe our approach of employing social media technology to accomplish research while being socially distanced. The description of how this process took place is an important part of our story of connecting and finding meaning during the pandemic. This section also serves as a methodological treatment for those who might be interested in doing interviews on social media with participants not accustomed to using these forms of technology.

Social distancing interviewing: Coping with technology

"Can you get your granddaughter to set you up on Skype?" I ask, after I explain to Jerry what this platform will allow us to do.

"I'll try, but my granddaughter isn't coming over much because she doesn't want to expose me to the virus."

"That's okay. There's no rush."

A few days later, Jerry's granddaughter opens a Skype account for him, and we make a connection while she sits beside him. This is the first time we've connected in this way; before, all our interactions have been face-to-face, or by phone or email. We both are thrilled to be able to observe each other as we talk; the visuals and nonverbals enliven the discussion.

"My granddaughter also showed me how to do messenger," Jerry says proudly.

We make a date to do the interview on Skype in a few days and I send him a list of questions to ponder. Though Jerry emails and googles regularly, I am apprehensive about whether he will be able to handle a new technology without assistance. Though I have used Skype frequently in the past to communicate with others, I have not done interviews before on social media. I need to find out how to record in Skype, and I want to explore how best to have our conversation transcribed. Is there an automatic transcription program that might assist us? Wanting to be prepared when our interview begins, I spend a few days researching the possibilities.

When I skype Jerry at our appointed time, I get a message that he is not online. I call him and he tells me he has been knocked off Skype for security reasons and has to input his information again. As he attempts to follow the instructions, he has difficulty deciphering the scrambled letters and numbers he has to identify to show he is not a robot.

"I have put in what I see 50 times, for two hours," he says.

His frustration and anxiety are palpable and I worry about his heart.

"Jerry, I also have trouble identifying those scrambled characters. Really, we can drop it. This interview is not that important."

"Yes it is," he says. "I want to do it."

"Let's try messenger," I suggest.

Our trial run on messenger is successful, and we are delighted with the quality of the sound and visuals. When I research how to record our conversation there, I discover that I can record only short segments by holding down a button with my finger. This won't work for a long interview.

Many phone calls later, I ask Jerry to try the Zoom platform, which I have used in the past. Zoom seems straight forward: I will send him an invitation and he can follow the prompts. Once we are online together, I assume I can help him with any problems he might have. I call him on his home phone, and instruct him to go to his email on his cell phone and find the invitation. Not accustomed to thinking of his phone as a computer, he insists he must use his laptop to click on the URL. When he does, we connect. But his computer is old, the picture is fuzzy, and it doesn't have a built-in microphone. I am disappointed that Zoom does not work for us, but wanting the technology to be as anxiety free as possible, I do not push him to try to connect on his cell.

"I'll try to get my granddaughter to help me," Jerry says, sounding defeated.

"Not to worry. If she doesn't come by, I have a backup plan."

A few days later I call Jerry again. Since he has gotten no help, I tell him that we will connect by messenger so we can at least see each other as we talk.

"I will place my portable voice recorder close to my phone and audio record what we say. We can't record and save the video, but I can record and save our conversation."

Our trial run works well. Then I do more research on automatic transcribing, spending a day learning how to use "TunestoTube" to convert my mp4 audio file to a file that can be put on YouTube so that I can use YouTube's closed caption transcription. When I run into myriad problems, including a length limitation, I turn to Audacity to shorten the tapes. When I finally get the closed captioning on YouTube to work, the automatic transcript is muddled with so many mistakes it is unusable. Editing the automatic transcription I then get from Scribie, another automatic transcription program I try, consumes as much time as it would have taken to do all the transcribing myself. I guess Jerry and I both have a lot to learn about pursuing this work long distance in the most efficient way. Days later, I write our story from the seventy-minute interview and from emails that Jerry and I pass back and forth as I ask for clarification on some issues we discussed. Finally I send him a rough draft. Understanding that I have pushed Jerry about as far as I can on learning new technology, I resist suggesting working with track changes in Microsoft Word on in Google Docs editor. Instead he sends me suggested changes by email and we then discuss the draft during a phone call.

The interview

"I think we're set to go then if you're ready," I say to Jerry, when his bottom jaw fills up the messenger frame.

"I'm ready."

"Can you hold your phone up higher so I can see your whole face?"

"It hurts my hand to hold up my arms. I get tired."

"Try to rest your elbows on the chair."

"It's April 13th, 2020, and I'm interviewing Jerry Rawicki," I say into the recorder.

"Jerry, I'm going to ask you questions about the pandemic. Overall, I am interested in how your experience now relates to your experience during the Holocaust, the similarities and differences, and how you might use coping mechanisms you learned then for now. We will take it one question at a time, okay?"

"Okay, just try to talk slow and loud, but don't yell at me."

I laugh. "You tell me if I'm not talking slowly or loud enough."

"Right now, it's fine. Go ahead."

Worrying as preparation for action

"Begin by talking about your experience during the pandemic."

"It's not much of an experience, really. You can't go anywhere. I can't go anywhere. Of course, I'm not complaining, because I am very comfortable here. I can read, I can write. The Holocaust is always superimposed on the pandemic and the pandemic makes me think about the Holocaust. I know everybody has been affected by the pandemic, but my nerves are on edge. I'm just about ready to jump out of my skin."

"Are your nerves worse now during the pandemic than they have been previously?"

"Yes, the pandemic has me very worried. I think about it all the time."

"What about it bothers you the most?"

"The unknown. I don't know what's going to happen and not knowing makes me imagine all kinds of things. I am seeing in my mind's eye scenes of the Holocaust when we did without food and necessities. I know I shouldn't be comparing the two because the privation and the problems now and those that we had during the Holocaust are diametrically different. But who knows. This situation we're in might all change for the worst. That's what I'm worried about."

"You are worried about things getting much worse than they are now?" I repeat.

"Yes in form and intensity. I can only speculate and that gets me down."

"Do you ever think about anything positive happening as a result of the pandemic?"

"It's a funny thing that you mention this. Just today, a friend sent me a video that suggested that lowering pollution, by reducing the use of the automobile, is a positive byproduct. The pollution all over the world has decreased. And the pollution kills more people than the pandemic probably will."

"And car accidents and crime are down," I say. "Do you think there could be any positive outcomes in terms of people's values?"

"Maybe the most positive thing will be that people will work together and the polarization in our country will be mitigated. Maybe countries also will start to cooperate to the betterment of humanity."

"Maybe people won't be as greedy as they are now, or perhaps they will find more meaning in relationships and realize how important their loved ones are to them," I add.

"Yes, maybe people will rethink the meaning of life. Is money important? Is fame important? Really the most important concern is your health and your family's wellbeing."

I think, but don't say, that this response might be more complicated for those under considerable economic pressure.

"I wonder why we tend to concentrate on the negative things, and worry about how much worse it all might get," I do say, to stay with the thread.

"You're talking to me and I'm a worry wart. Even in good times, I always think of the things that can go wrong. Maybe this is because of what I went through in the Holocaust. But I always say that not to think about things that can happen would be shortsighted. We cannot put our head in the sand. Especially during times like now, we have to think about what is going to happen; that is how we prepare ourselves."

"It sounds like for you that worry is a way to prepare."

Jerry nods. "It is. For example, I worry about my health and I take eleven pills a day. I have to prepare and make sure I have enough medication."

"I understand that. Did you worry during the Holocaust? Would you have called yourself a worrier when you were that young boy trying to escape? Was preparation then important?"

"I tried to prepare myself when I could. For example, I held onto the clean shirt when I escaped through the hole in the wall of the Warsaw Ghetto so that I could put it on and pass for Polish, rather than being identified as a Jew from the ghetto (Ellis & Rawicki, 2019). But in most situations, I didn't have time to prepare. I just tried to survive."

"Isn't there a difference between preparing and worrying?"

"In my case, worrying stimulated me to prepare."

"It sounds like you think it is your responsibility to worry. That if you aren't worried right now, you wouldn't be being responsible. You wouldn't be doing what you have to do."

"Exactly. And it's important because I'm in that age group that is in more danger than younger people. So, for example, if I wasn't worried about what happens, I would go out now to the grocery store or other appointments. But that would be a foolish thing to do."

"I'm with you," I agree, nodding my head. "I'm in the vulnerable age range too, and so I don't go out. Besides, I don't want to infect others, in case I'm a carrier without symptoms. These are choices we all have to make."

Making choices

"This morning when I woke up, my back hurt," I begin. "Art had an appointment with the chiropractor for tomorrow, but he said he was afraid to go. And so I thought, 'Well, maybe I will go in his place.' I felt justified since I was in pain. But I decided not to go. If Art didn't want to expose himself that way, then I shouldn't either. Because if I got the virus, then I'd also probably give it to him. So although Art said I should make my own decision, it didn't feel like the decision was mine to make alone. These are interesting choices confronting us."

"This is what is happening to us now," Jerry responds. "It's a pandemic and it can go on and on. And if it does, we'll have more of these choices to confront. For example, maybe there will come a time that we can't be on the computer together like we are doing now."

"That would be awful."

"This is what scares me, the unknown," Jerry repeats.

"What kinds of choices are you having to make other than not going out?" I ask

"In addition to the obvious—that we must endure what has befallen us—the question is how we can fill the void. I meditate now more often and deeply than usual, and listen to more music. And I'm trying to finish writing my novel though the distractions of the political situation get in my way. I'm trying unsuccessfully to stay away from TV, and hating myself for not being able to shake off my obsession with politics. In that regard, I can identify with heroin and meth users. Basically, I'm trying to stay healthy. That is my choice."

"What are you doing to stay healthy, other than staying inside, meditating, and listening to music?" I ask.

"Diet is something I'm very much concerned with, given my congestive heart failure and history of lymphoma. I may think of fancy restaurants, but Campbell's chicken soup does nicely."

I smile and think that chicken soup does nicely for me as well. "Anything else?"

"My passion once upon a time was tennis. As recently as two months ago, I supplanted that by walking in the Publix parking lot when I went shopping. Now even that is out of my reach, so instead I exercise during my shower time, doing scaled down calisthenics."

"What do you miss most now while sheltering in place?"

"Of course, as I've said, I miss not going out, even by way of Lyft. I miss shopping for myself, having lunch with friends. That was all abbreviated naturally as the years kept advancing but now it feels for me, as it does for many, like being in jail. Of course I'm trying to compensate by pretending the old normal, rather than the new normal we find ourselves in, is still in place. But if nothing else, seeing my car sitting idly waiting to be disposed of reminds of an era going by, my personal fin de siècle, sad but true."

I wonder if this imprisonment feels like a life sentence to him, but I don't want to dwell on the end of life. Instead, I say, "I'm reminded of how different things are now from when you were in the Holocaust. There your choices were different from deciding whether you go to the store."

"Indeed, then it was all about surviving each moment."

Comparing the COVID-19 Pandemic to the Holocaust

"Does the pandemic make you think more about the Holocaust than you normally do?"

"Yes, it does. Well, I always think about that time, but now I'm thinking about the Holocaust as a background to determine how bad things are now. Though the discomfort and the anxiety I feel are unpleasant, compared to the Holocaust, they are minor. I know the pandemic might continue, but I don't think it will ever assume the dimensions of the Holocaust. In some ways, the Holocaust works as a matrix against which I consider things. I say to myself, 'If I survived the Bodzentyn ghetto and severe starvation, I surely can survive the grocery stores not having enough bread or cake.'"

"Or toilet paper," I say, and then wait.

"In Bodzentyn and the Warsaw Ghetto, life was predictable in that if I went out I would be killed. I had a target on my back. But this pandemic is a maybe situation. If I go out, maybe I will be infected, maybe I won't."

"That's an interesting comparison. There you knew that people were trying to kill you, and if you gave them a chance you would be killed. Now you might escape the virus or you might not. It's an invisible enemy. Right?"

"That's correct."

"How would you compare your feelings now to those you had during the Holocaust?"

"My feelings during the Holocaust depended on the circumstance. For example, are we talking about when as a 10-year-old boy I listened to Hitler's updates, or when I arrived in the Ghetto in Bodzentyn, or somewhere in between? Are we talking about the fear I felt when I saw a gendarme at the end of the street and ran to hide? Or about my feelings of sadness leaving Bodzentyn when I realized I might never see my mother again? Or the euphoria when I managed to squeeze myself through the bricks and exit the Warsaw Ghetto?"

"Yes, I can see that my question is complicated by circumstance. But how would you describe your feelings now? You have mentioned several times your increased anxiety. Can you say more about that? Do you feel all those other feelings like sadness, euphoria, fear? Of course I realize feelings are experienced differently when you are 93 from when you are 16, but I'm wondering if you have any insight about what it feels like to be 93 in terms of emotionality and dealing with this pandemic."

"Though not comparable to what I felt during the Holocaust, my anxiety now is heightened to the absolute nth. The virus as it now intersects with politics devastates me. I think of the future and what it may look like if Trump succeeds for a second term. As we talked about earlier, I admit my preoccupation with the nightly updates borders on obsession and it all stays with me. It depresses me."

"Don't you take an anti-depressant or anti-anxiety drug?"

"I did, but because of my heart, my doctor took me off of it. Too bad that I've always pooh poohed shrinks."

"We'll come back to Trump, I promise. But let's look at other things that might factor into your feelings. For example, I'm wondering if the images of the pandemic that you see on TV affect you, and if so, how."

"They do. For example, yesterday I saw rows of caskets and people digging graves. I'm not sure where it was."

"New York, I think."

"Yes, that's it. They found unidentified poor people in the street and buried them in a large rectangular grave. It made me think about how I used to dig graves in Bodzentyn. Not rectangular ones, just holes in the ground. And I recalled the dead bodies in the Warsaw Ghetto. The photos reminded me about finding a body on the street in Bodzentyn. I wondered if it was somebody I knew."

"That's an intense image, Jerry. It makes me shiver."

"The pictures of the vacant city streets also affect me. They are like ghost towns and remind me of the bubonic plague when things looked barren."

"Are you having a lot of dreams?"

"I don't dream much. When I do it's hard to remember what they are about. And even when I remember, I have no idea how to interpret them. I don't think I ever dreamed about the Holocaust."

"Really? You never have?"

"Not that I remember, though I daydream about the Holocaust all the time."

"You're not dreaming in your sleep about the pandemic either?"

"No."

"I don't either, actually. Are you sleeping well?"

"Yes, very well. I take Turmeric every night and that helps."

"Good, sleep is important for your health. Did you worry about viruses and contagious diseases during the Holocaust?"

"Oh yes. Typhus was rampant. The pandemic has made me wonder why I didn't get typhus from the close quarters I shared in that storefront in Bodzentyn with my mother and sister, who had Typhus. I recall now that when I left Bodzentyn for Warsaw, I was worried because I didn't feel good. Now I wonder if I might actually have had typhus then. Even if I did, I didn't have it to the extent of my sister for whom it was deadly. And maybe I didn't feel right just because I was depressed from taking care of her and then having to leave her and my mother."

"Sometimes I wonder why I survived," Jerry continues. "I'm not a religious person, but I am spiritual and I meditate. I think now that I must be here to tell the story of what happened during the Holocaust. Not because I am a writer or a person of knowledge or a philosopher, but maybe in my own little sphere, maybe I'm supposed to live to contribute something. I feel the same way now about the pandemic."

"Yes, I think that telling the story of your experience has become your purpose in life in many ways."

"I say to myself that there are so many people around me who died during the Holocaust and they were better people than me. This is what makes me think that anybody on this planet who survived should be able to give something back, not material things necessarily, but maybe things that are just as important to meaningful living."

"I like that, Jerry. Do you think that you have wisdom from your experience during the Holocaust that you might offer to help you or others during the pandemic or even help yourself?"

"No, I don't think it is wisdom. I think that when it comes to coping with what we have now that my feelings are a product of my experiences in the Holocaust. Of course being on lockdown and confined to the house is different from being confined to a storefront with ten other people and forbidden to step outside under the penalty of death. Right now, it is difficult to imagine this virus would be really destructive and dystopian, or to think that we might have hunger in Tampa or St. Petersburg the same way we had it in Bodzentyn or Warsaw. But if we did, I think having gone through hunger, confinement, and disease as I did that I might be able to cope better than a person who was never exposed to anything like that."

"How about psychologically? Do you think you're more prepared psychologically?"

"When I imagine something beyond our pandemic, something like bubonic plague or the Spanish flu, I know that psychologically I would be completely done in. That kind of hunger would kill me physically as well as psychologically. I don't think I would be able to live another day or another hour if I had to face anything like what I faced during the Holocaust. Of course, that's partly due to my age. When I was 16 or 18, I could withstand many, many more pressures than I can now. If it came to this point, I would just say, I don't want to go through it."

"Yes, certainly your age is a factor, as is mine. I don't think I could survive hunger. I've never experienced hunger or thought much about it, except in hearing your story about starvation. But I have found myself thinking about the possibility that something might happen to our food chain. That's frightening. I find myself reading every article having to do with food or grocery stores. I think that's the strongest of my fears. Do you understand people hoarding food now?"

"Yes, of course. They are hoarding it because they are afraid of the future and for their physical wellbeing. People are afraid they won't be able to do without, just as you mentioned. I guess a few hoard things to sell later, but that's an exception, and I guess you can hoard to a level that is pathological, such as with toilet paper."

"Did you think about toilet paper during the Holocaust?"

"I didn't and I don't remember much about toilets. In Bodzentyn we had an outhouse when we were confined to the storefront, and I remember that my mother urged my two sisters to use it. They were afraid to go because they feared men would watch them. In the transfer camp before taking us to Bodzentyn, the Germans forced us to relieve ourselves in the open fields. But otherwise, I don't remember thinking about hygiene during the Holocaust. I don't know if I took baths or whether I had soap. I certainly never had toothpaste. That's why my teeth are as bad as they are now. It just wasn't something I was thinking about. Most of the time, I was like an animal responding to emergencies. I watch National Geographic quite a bit, and I see how I reacted to danger just like the animals do."

"Do you think you were more of a feeling than thinking person during the Holocaust?"

"It is hard to consider feeling and thinking in tandem though considering them separately is not useful either. The best answer I have is that my feeling and thinking depended on time, circumstances, and location. For example, in the cellar in the Warsaw Ghetto as I subsisted on rotten potatoes, I acted and felt like an animal. That lasted through being caught and led toward the Umshlagplatz, where I would either be killed or sent off to a camp. But when I escaped and got into Warsaw proper, my thinking brain kicked in and I thought about changing into a clean shirt and finding my sister. So my feeling and thinking during the Holocaust acted independently or in concert depending on my psyche at a time, homo sapiens or animal. Now, during this pandemic, without the physical terror I experienced during the Holocaust, I can feel and think like a normal person."

Connecting and making meaning during the pandemic

"We've talked about how your experience of the Holocaust has influenced your experience now and affected how you cope, and about how your experiences might have differed at age 16 from your experiences now at age 93," I write to Jerry in an email. "But we haven't talked about how your experience of the pandemic at 93 years old might differ from the experience of younger people. How might your worries be different from a younger person in terms of thinking about the future, for example?"

Jerry doesn't respond for a day, which is unusual.

> Then he writes, "You are asking me to compare my experiences and concerns with those of younger people. I wish I knew what they think and how they feel, but I don't and nothing comes to mind that I can add."

Jerry's email makes me think about the difficulty of some of the questions I have posed to him: asking a 93-year-old man to reflect on his emotional experiences almost 80 years before; asking him to recall how it all felt so long ago, as though his feelings were monochrome and not dependent on each situation he found himself in; asking him to talk about his feelings now, when most of us would have trouble deciphering and separating any feeling we have from the overarching sensation of anxiety that permeates so many of our lives; and then asking him to compare his feelings to those of someone much younger. If it's difficult to figure out what we ourselves are feeling during these uncertain times, how would we know what others are feeling, especially when, as older people, we are isolated and not interacting much with anyone, much less younger people? I don't know how much younger people are worrying, for example. Are they, like Jerry at 18, able to stand more pressures than we, in our later years, are able to endure? Are their worries more about finances and their economic futures than about their health? Jerry doesn't know, and neither do I.

I would have trouble answering the questions I'm asking. This makes me, as a researcher, question my questions (Bochner, personal correspondence). As I do, I get more insight into why it is so difficult to write about our emotional experience, including my own, during the pandemic in any meaningful way.

> "I am interested in what gives our lives meaning," I say to Jerry, still wanting to say something meaningful about our experience. "And the significance of connections and relationships, especially now when we are isolated and sheltering in place."
>
> "Connecting with others has always been important to me. I am very gregarious. I've always loved getting together with friends. But even before the pandemic, getting together had become more difficult because I'm not as ambulatory as I was. I told you that I gave my granddaughter my car?"
>
> "Yes, you told me. Was that hard?"
>
> "No, because I already had made up my mind not to drive. And I can always call an Uber."
>
> "During the Holocaust, you didn't have a car or Uber, or access to the telephone. You certainly didn't have email friends as you do now, or access to the internet. Other than a message or letter that at rare times might reach you, you had no contact with those from whom you were separated. Though we now have to shelter in place and can't visit physically, what's different now is that we can connect by technology, as in our case, with messenger. Can you speak to that?"

"I am thankful for the technology because it is wonderful. But it has its lows as well as highs. For example, Facebook. If it was up to me I would cut it completely. But I do like getting pictures of my grandchildren, which is why I got on it in the first place. But then I think of the millions of people who are using their Facebook for political or selfish reasons to create nothing but a cesspool."

"Do you get on Facebook and read other people's messages?"

"I try, but I'm completely lost on the Facebook in terms of navigating it. I put things on about Trump occasionally, but I really want the world to read my posts. I care less about being read by friends who have the same political leanings as I do. My son Andy told me I'd have to have more friends to accomplish that. So I tried what he told me to do and I ended up befriending a stranger in Montana."

Jerry and I laugh.

"If I see something important, I do add my comments," Jerry continues. "So in that respect, the Facebook is helping me to express myself politically. But as hard as I try, the negative feelings stay with me. Even though the posting should be a positive outlet for me, just the opposite occurs: it depresses me."

"Throughout this interview, and really during the whole time I've known you, politics has been meaning-making in your life and yet it's also your Achilles heel in a way. You keep up with what is going on as much as anybody I know. It adds to your life in that it engages your passion. And yet at the same time, you talk about being obsessed by it and how upset that makes you."

"That is true. The thing that bothers me most about the pandemic is how it is politicized by Trump. Until a few days ago I listened each day to Trump's two or more hours of so-called briefings. I don't know how I endured it. Now I rely on what I hear the following day from cable news. Trump spouts the same platitudes and garbage every day. He is imbecilic and repetitious."

I nod and sigh.

"I think often about the paper you and I did on Trump (Ellis & Rawicki, 2018). There we made a case for the similarities between Trump and Hitler."

"You mean how they both basked in the glow of the crowds on their victory tours and how they mesmerized and aroused their supporters?"

"Exactly and repeated big lies, the more outrageous the better…"

"And generated slogans."

"Even worse, Trump makes his reputation by defaming others, never admitting wrong or accepting blame," I add. "And picks an enemy, like Hilary or Obama, and never lets up on them."

"I go on Facebook feeling it is my obligation to tell the world of the danger we are in and what it portends for the immediate future," Jerry says. "I don't know if you followed all my Facebook posts in the last few weeks. Often the kind of thing I say is then mentioned in the newspapers the next day. And a few people like my posts so that all makes my heart happy because I see there are people, other than my friends, who think like you and I do."

"I know. I get that kind of response on Facebook. It does feel good. I hear what you're saying about the negative aspects of Facebook. I try to go through those argumentative posts quickly. But I have a wonderful group of more than 500 friends and acquaintances now on Facebook, and almost without exception, they view the world the way I do. Now some people argue that it is not good to surround yourself only with like-minded folks. I know that you, for example, listen to Fox and MSNBC for various opinions and then make up your own mind. But. Jerry, I just can't listen to Fox. I'd rather spend my time reading the articles my Facebook friends post and the newspapers I receive each day. Having a community of like-minded people soothes my soul and makes my life feel meaningful in this time of hate-filled lies and animosity."

"I also like it when I get likes, especially from people who I know have been Trump supporters in the past."

"So then you understand a bit about what I am talking about." Jerry nods. "I especially liked your post on April 14th," I say, "the one that elicited several comments."

Pulling up the post on my laptop screen, I read it aloud.

Monday night Trump's coronavirus update turned infomercial political rally was for lack of a more horrid word an abomination. If that was not egregious enough, Fox, the shadow White House, doubled up on it just a few minutes ago through its marquee daily 'Outnumbered' farce. There in the splendor of his office, the vice president and the cabal of the rest of his willing accomplices sprawled apart as per the President's guidelines, six feet apart, their angelic smiles illuminating the theater of the absurd. As the curtain went up and the president encouraged his guests to share with the American People, meaning his base, their stories of their miraculous recovery, it was difficult to abstain from reaching for a vial of hydroxychloroquine. What did we have to lose? Please understand, my sardonic language is not to make light of the tragedy that's besetting us now as we speak. Quite the opposite, I'm raising alarms to a pandemic that is not the only pestilence that threatens our live; the other one is the president and his cohorts who unabashedly, brazenly and cruelly tinker with our senses and sensibilities. I said or implied it before and I'll say it again, It is not fashionable, at least not yet, to talk about legacies of Stalin and his Beria, Hitler and his Goebbels, and their Gulags and Death Camps, but it all started with megalomania, psychotic narcissism, devilish cunning, mass rallies, pies in the sky, pathological lying and unmitigated gall. I was twelve years old in 1939 and when my parents turned up the radio to listen to Hitler's nightly harangue, I heard it all. Now as I type this, I remember it as it were yesterday.

"When I post things on Facebook like what you just read, I hope I am providing something useful," Jerry says.

"You are Jerry. I think people pay attention to your posts partly because they are wise, but also because you lived through the Holocaust. Readers want to know what you think and perhaps it gives them hope to remember that you lived through a time much worse than we are experiencing now. I think readers will feel the same way about what you have to say in this interview."

"Do you think we have come up with something worthwhile here?"

"I hope so. We'll work on the text together, after I transcribe it and write a draft. This doesn't have to be our final word."

"I always like to talk to you and be interviewed by you. It keeps my mind working."

"Being able to experience each other, to see expressions and faces in addition to voices, to be aware of the nonverbal, that made me feel we had a significant visit. Our connection was deeper than we would have had on a phone conversation. What about you?"

"It was the difference between day and night. I can't even compare it," Jerry replies. "And I could hear every word, I'm comfortable with my arms resting on the arm chair, and I'm not even tired. Maybe we can do it again. It helps me to talk with you."

"It helps me too. I feel connected to you and like we're doing something meaningful together. Connecting and finding a way to engage in meaningful activity—two important ways to cope with our anxieties, fears, and sense of isolation during the pandemic."

Note

1. In particular, I find myself captivated by the personal story that Chris Cuomo tells on CNN each night. Reporting from his basement, he emotionally describes fever, chills, fatigue, and hallucinations he experiences while having COVID-19 (Cuomo, April 13, 2020). His biggest fear is realized when his wife comes down with the virus, and then his fourteen-year-old son. "I'm scared by the potential of this," he says, and later talks about the mental issues he is having as a result of the virus (April 24, 2020). If Chris can get it, then I can too, I think. We all can.

   Again on CNN, a father—a retired physician—talks lovingly and without tears about his daughter, who was head of an emergency department at a Manhattan hospital. She got the virus and then later committed suicide. "She tried to do her job, and it killed her," her father said (New York Post, April 28, 2020). I take it all in, the grief of the father, the loss of this young forty-nine-year-old emergency doctor who gave so much. It feels like the least I can do. Then I imagine, 'What if it were me or someone I loved?'

References

Cuomo, C. (2020, April 13). *Covid-19 update: I can't shake my fever.* Video file. https://www.youtube.com/watch?v=P3U1ufVvr3U

Cuomo, C. (2020, April 24). *Chris Cuomo on Covid-19 Recovery: Dr. Sanjay Gupta's coronavirus podcast for April 24.* Podcast. https://www.cnn.com/2020/04/24/health/chris-cuomo-sanjay-gupta-podcast-transcript-april-24-wellness/index.html

Ellis, C. (1993). There are survivors": Telling a story of a sudden death. *The Sociological Quarterly, 34*(4), 711–730. https://doi.org/10.1111/j.1533-8525.1993.tb00114.x

Ellis, C. (1995, 2018). *Final negotiations: A story of love, loss, and chronic illness.* Philadelphia, Pa:Temple University Press.

Ellis, C. (1996). Maternal connections. In C. Ellis & A. P. Bochner (Eds.), *Composing ethnography: Alternative forms of qualitative writing.* (pp. 240–243). AltaMira Press.

Ellis, C. (2002). Shattered Lives: Making sense of September 11th and its aftermath. *Journal of Contemporary Ethnography, 31*(4), 375–410. https://doi.org/10.1177/0891241602031004001

Ellis, C., & Patti, C. (2014). With heart: Compassionate interviewing and storytelling with Holocaust survivors. *Storytelling, Self, Society, 10*(1), 389–414.

Ellis, C., & Rawicki, J. (2013). Collaborative witnessing of survival during the Holocaust: An exemplar of relational autoethnography. *Qualitative Inquiry, 19*(5), 366–380. https://doi.org/10.1177/1077800413479562

Ellis, C., & Rawicki, J. (2018). Remembering the past/Anticipating the future: A professor from the white working class talks with a survivor of the Holocaust about our troubled world. *Qualitative Inquiry, 24*(5), 323–337. https://doi.org/10.1177/1077800417741387

Ellis, C., & Rawicki, J. (2019). The clean shirt: A flicker of hope in despair. *Journal of Contemporary Ethnography, 48*(1), 3–15. https://doi.org/10.1177/0891241617696809

New York Post (April 28, 2020). (*Top New York City ER doctor commits suicide, shaken by coronavirus onslaught.* Retrieved from https://www.foxnews.com/health/top-manhattan-er-doc-commits-suicide-shaken-coronavirus-onslaught

Noonan, P. (2020). What comes after the coronavirus storm? We'll eventually get to a safe harbor, but we'll find we're a changed country. *Wall Street Journal* (Opinion). (April 23). https://www.wsj.com/articles/what-comes-after-the-coronavirus-storm-11587684752

Rawicki, J., & Ellis, C. (2011). Lechem hara (bad bread) Lechem tov (good bread): Depravity and nobility during the Holocaust. *Qualitative Inquiry, 17*(2), 155–157.

Impact of COVID-19 on Athletes and Coaches, and Their Values in Japan: Repercussions of Postponing the Tokyo 2020 Olympic and Paralympic Games

Kanako Taku and Hirokazu Arai

ABSTRACT
On 24 March 2020, an announcement was made that the Tokyo 2020 Olympic and Paralympic games would be postponed until 2021 due to the coronavirus pandemic. Athletes and their coaches have experienced a wide spectrum of emotional and cognitive reactions such as disappointment, frustration, confusion, and relief, to name a few. The current article aimed to summarize the athletes' and coaches' reactions related to the repercussions triggered by the postponement of the Tokyo 2020 Olympic and Paralympic Games in Japan, and discuss how the values of sports and athletes have or are likely to be changed.

On March 12th 2020, the Olympic flame was lit at the site of ancient Olympia in Greece to prepare for the Tokyo 2020 Olympic and Paralympic Games. The news also reported that, in Greece, people were unfortunately not allowed to attend the flame lighting ceremony because of the coronavirus outbreak, which we have seen spreading around the world. This happened a day after March 11th, the day that has a special meaning for Japanese people, since the triple disaster (i.e., earthquake, tsunami, and nuclear power plan meltdown) hit the northeast coast of Japan on March 11th 2011, where nearly 16,000 people lost their lives. The flame could have been the ideal symbol for recovery, reconstruction, and resilience for, at least some people in Japan, especially in the devastated communities, even though there are still more than 47,000 people that are displaced as of May 2020, nine years after the disaster.

Despite the concerns of the coronavirus pandemic, a plane left Tokyo to pick up the torch from Greece so the relay could start in the area where the most severe damage occurred by the tsunami in 2011. The flame in fact arrived in Japan on March 20th 2020. The flame was placed in a lantern while an increasing number of cases of coronavirus were being reported on the daily basis. On March 22nd, the media reported that the International Olympic Committee (IOC) would make an announcement in the "next four weeks" of the game status. While the IOC had not yet rendered their final decision on whether the games would proceed or not, Canada announced that they would not send any athletes to compete. On March 24th, the IOC and the Tokyo Organizing Committee announced that the Tokyo 2020 Olympic and Paralympic Games would be postponed until 2021. It was only two days before the day that the relay was supposed to start. Approximately 10,000 runners ranging from 12 years old to 94 years old were supposed to relay the torch starting on March 26th to the day of opening ceremony, on July 24th.

This article aimed to keep the record of our observations related to the repercussions due to the postponement of Tokyo 2020 Olympic and Paralympic Games by focusing on its historical background, athletes and their coaches, and the values of athletes and sports in Japan.

Background

Japan previously experienced the cancelation of the Olympic and Paralympic Games that were scheduled to happen in 1940 due to World War II. Twenty-four years later, in 1964, Japan hosted the summer Olympic and Paralympic games and considered them as an opportunity to broadcast how the country, Japan, recovered and experienced economic growth after World War II. People who remembered the passion and excitement that the community created in the Tokyo 1964 Olympic and Paralympic Games in their childhood are now in their 50s, 60s, and older. One such person is Mr. Hiroshi Kondo, aged 72, who was selected to relay the torch in 1964 but canceled due to a typhoon, and this time, he was then selected again to relay the torch for the Olympic and Paralympic Games on May 25th 2020. Yet, we now know it will once again be canceled. Another person, aged 63, told us how happy and proud he was when he was selected to relay the torch for the 2020 Games. Since he is 63 years old, he knows this is most likely to be his last opportunity to participate in the Olympic and Paralympic games in Japan as a torch runner. Since he was assigned to relay the torch at the end of June in 2020, he had already started physical training so that he could hold the torch to a certain height, as well as purchased equipment, clothes, and shoes. He was therefore disappointed when the postponement was announced. Moreover, given that he was selected to relay the torch as a representative of his company, his employees were even more disappointed, as this could have been a great opportunity to advertise their company (Note: It is prohibited to wear a company shirt but allowed to announce on the company website, which increases public attention, leading to indirect advertising effect). Even though the Tokyo Olympic and Paralympic Games cannot be guaranteed to take place in 2021 and he may not be selected as a torch runner, he said he is trying to maintain motivation.

Another symbolic person is the current Japanese Prime Minister, Shinzo Abe, whose grandfather was also the prime minister at the time of the Tokyo 1964 Olympic and Paralympic Games. In 1964, the Olympic torch was carried and used to light the Olympic cauldron by a person who was born in Hiroshima on August 6th 1945, the day that the atomic bomb was dropped on the city during World War II. The Olympic and Paralympic Games have historically been considered as an opportunity to unite people, foster diversity, and demonstrate the glory of each country that sends athletes who represent their country. Perhaps because of these backgrounds, coupled with historical and religious characteristics that Japanese culture holds, Japanese Deputy Prime Minister, Taro Aso, remarked that it is the cursed Olympics. The postponement of the 2020 Tokyo Olympic and Paralympic Games has shaken the expectations of the public and their values to the core.

Athletes

A direct impact was made on the athletes and players who have trained for the 2020 Tokyo Olympic and Paralympic Games for a long time. For some, the announcement of postponement automatically meant retirement and the eternal loss of opportunity. For instance, Tom Ransley, a double Olympic medalist on the British rowing team, announced his retirement. The Rio Olympic silver medalist, Eddie Dawkins, also announced his retirement from tack cycling. For others, however, the postponement merely indicates the temporal shift of timing and quick adjustment to optimize their peak so they can use it as an extended chance to further improve their performance or recover from injuries they might have endured. Overall, these players maintain optimistic and positive attitudes. And yet for others, it means an existential crisis. For instance, it used to be reasonable for athletes to focus on their own physical and mental condition while training, because they were able to assume that the schedule of official games, such as Olympic and Paralympic Games, will happen as they were scheduled. The athletes were able to allocate their energy and time for training, practice, or therapies, and control their motivation to adjust their peak, because again they were certain that the games would happen. However, this assumption has been disrupted. The COVID-19 pandemic fundamentally changed the players' cognitive assumptions in that they will no longer take these events and schedules for granted. From now on, it may be that, in the back of their minds, no matter how they prepare, the game may be postponed or canceled. In general, we heard that most players, whether they like it or not, accept the postponement but strongly hope that nothing will lead to cancelation of Tokyo Olympic and Paralympic Games.

Another aspect that was lost is the daily, weekly, monthly, and annual routine, affecting the mental and physical status of players. When the triple disaster happened in 2011, many players lost their daily routine for training as well, and yet, the impact remained localized. The impact of the nuclear power plant accident was invisible, and yet, there were many parts of Japan that were far enough from Fukushima prefecture that allowed athletes to continue their training. The spread of COVID-19 has not only forced nearly every training location to shut down, but also forces players to stay home. Social distancing precautions enacted to slow the spread of COVID-19 have affected not only the Tokyo Olympic and Paralympic games, but all other games as well, including the cancelation of qualification tournaments. These changes have increased a sense of uncertainty, confusion, and frustration, and made it difficult to set a series of concrete goals.

In addition, because of limited opportunities to leave the house and do intensive and systematic training, when the players were allowed to practice for a shorter period of time, they tend to overwork to maximize the impact, which could increase the likelihood of injuries, which in turn, could lead even more to a sense of doubt and frustration. Limited interactions with teammates, coaches, and others may make athletes even more anxious due to further uncertainty. Due to social distancing mandates, more players increase their use of social networking services (SNS) to connect with society. Although strong support from fans and the community could give the players a sense of connectedness, unity, and pride, it could make them feel more anxious and overwhelmed.

Furthermore, athletes who heavily rely on the Olympic and Paralympic games, especially those with less visible sports and para-athletes, often have side jobs to support their lives. Without knowing the exact schedules or the additional funding that may be allocated, some may need to increase their workload or, on the contrary, have already lost their job and/or sponsorship. Many players are concerned if the cost of their training and preparation for the Olympic and Paralympic Games could still be fully covered.

In addition, it has been pointed out that the COVID-19 pandemic has increased concerns for doping. Due to this pandemic, tests have been temporarily paused in many cases, giving some athletes the chances to consider trying performance-enhancing drugs, which in turn, increases the anxiety and doubt for the other competitive players who refrain from doping.

Furthermore, some players are concerned how medications they may need to take if they get infected by COVID-19 will be detected and judged due to the lack of reliable information.

Overall, due to restricted and challenging training environments around the globe, it would be challenging for players to maintain their best conditions, follow special diets, and work on the individualized tasks to break records and achieve a high level of performance at the prospective Tokyo Olympic and Paralympic Games. However, we also have observed athletes taking this as an opportunity to care for their wounds, strengthen themselves, and develop their creativity, such as using face masks to simulate high altitude physical training.

Coaches

Coaches and instructors were yet another group of people who were affected by the COVID-19 pandemic. There were, for example, some sports that had not yet selected their final members for Olympic and Paralympic Games. Several screening meetings and selection races/games were planned during the spring. There were short periods of time that these pre-selection games were postponed or canceled but the decisions for the actual Olympic and Paralympic Games were not made, therefore, trainers had a particular difficulty in coaching the players. Although the postponement of the Olympic and Paralympic Games were announced shortly after, the trainers needed to explore the most effective ways to coach the players under circumstances that they have never experienced. This pressure may also be associated with the collectivistic cultural characteristics of Japan, increasing a sense of responsibility. Since the Olympic and Paralympic Games will happen in their home country of Japan, it is more difficult to use defensive coping strategies like self-handicapping (e.g., situations will not allow them to make excuses such as "food was different," "confused because of the language barrier," "unable to show the best performance due to the jet lag," "weather was unfamiliar"). Japanese coaches may feel more constant pressure to get as many medals as possible due to proximate social pressure of home advantage. As increasing attention has been paid to athletes for the Tokyo Olympic and Paralympic Games, increasing opportunities to be on media, receive requests for interviews, connect with SNS (and the players are also more willing to do so). Similarly, as more companies sponsor athletes as a marketing strategy, the social impact of the way players communicate in public will ultimately affect whether the player will be selected as a member for Olympic and Paralympic Games. As these players receive financial support for their performance, the COVID-19 pandemic may prompt questions around guilt and fairness (e.g., "Without playing, do I deserve this?"). Coaches may now need to assist them to cope with these issues, help develop skills to use SNS or to appear in public, experiences which they themselves never experienced in their youth.

In addition, coaches are also affected by the pandemic directly. They may not be able to allocate enough time and energy to focus on their players' conditions, since they need to take care of themselves as well as their families. Coaches who are not directly involved in the Tokyo Olympic and Paralympic Games are also affected. For instance, the institutions such as All Japan High School Athletic Federation carefully arranged the games for youths outside of the weeks for the Olympic and Paralympic Games to avoid double-booking to make sure that the younger athletes will have an opportunity to watch the Olympic and Paralympic Games, which in turn made coaches of youth sports re-arrange their training schedules. Due to the current uncertain situation, coupled with continued cancelation or postponement of other local (e.g., city, prefectures) and national-level games, they too have faced difficulty in systematically scheduling their education and training their student athletes.

Values of Athletes and Sports

The COVID-19 crisis can be viewed from the perspective of trauma (Horesh & Brown, 2020), and is likely to be a turning point in the values of sports and athletes. Values give a sense of purpose, for the reasons why athletes compete, which in turn helps them set short-term and long-term career goals. On one hand, the meaning of values that society places on sports (i.e., societal values) have been challenged by the COVID-19 pandemic. On the other hand, the values each player holds (i.e., personal values) have also been shaken. These personal values may also be divided into terminal values and instrumental values, often measured by the Rokeach Value Survey (Johnston, 1995). Terminal values are concerned with end states of existence (e.g., social recognition such as "my ultimate purpose for playing sports is to become famous and recognized"), whereas instrumental values are concerned with modes of conduct (e.g., honesty such as "one thing that guides my principles is to be fair and honest").

These two values, that is, societal and the two aspects of personal values, may conflict with one another and there are players who struggle with between societal values (e.g., "athletes are supposed to make a full commitment for training and win for the country") and personal values (e.g., "my priority is to enjoy each moment regardless of the consequences"). It is difficult to stay motivated when one's values are shaken. Furthermore, players have developed and embraced these values because of how they construct their identity as an "athlete." As time goes by without training or competing, the athlete's sense of identity itself is also challenged. When it is difficult to hold a firm sense of identity as an athlete, they may seek for a rapid means of getting social support, such as SNS, as a psychological crutch. Due to social distancing, connecting with people around the globe on SNS may be helpful for an athlete, however, given that many athletes allow their SNS to be interactive, negative and harsh comments can also be directed toward them, which in turn, affects the values they hold in themselves and sports. In fact, sport fans are no longer passive receivers of value but rather can be active value co-creators, as pointed out by studies that focused on commercial values (e.g., Kolyperas et al., 2019; Woratschek et al., 2014).

Perhaps the collectivistic characteristics of Japanese culture accelerates each members' desires to "be needed" under conditions of uncertainty. One athlete told us that she wished she could be given some role she can play for a team so that she could lean on it without heavily ruminating the current situation.

Conclusions

Four years ago, there was a debate regarding how athletes and visitors would face risk of infection by the Zika virus during the Olympic and Paralympic Games in Rio de Janeiro (e.g., Warnke & Paul, 2016). Several players in fact chose not to attend the games due to the Zika virus. As many point out, we should have taken the impact more seriously and developed systems to cope with pandemic. The Olympic and Paralympic Games in Paris in 2024 have been scheduled regardless. If the Tokyo 2020 games take place in 2021, then there will only be 3 years until the Paris 2024 games, which will have its own repercussions. Some athletes may be able to perform better because they can apply their experiences in Tokyo 2020 to Paris 2024. It may add more pressure on athletes due to a shorter period of time between the games and some may start a new training schedule without taking enough of a break after the Tokyo Olympic and Paralympic Games. Furthermore, the Beijing Winter Olympic and Paralympic Games have been scheduled for February, 2022. Because the fiscal year in Japan starts on April 1and ends on March 31, there will be two Olympic and Paralympic games within the same fiscal year for Japanese people. This may affect the budgets that will be allocated to each athlete, team, sport, and game, which is also of great concern to the athletes and coaches.

Due to the uncertainty (i.e., Tokyo Olympic and Paralympic Games are currently postponed to 2021 and yet, it is not guaranteed to take place), it is plausible that most athletes will "wait" until the final decisions are made.

The debates and decisions of many sport games around the world being canceled have questioned the values of sports, by sending a message that sports are not essential for human survival. We would like to conclude this article by encouraging all of us to actively engage in and focus on what we can do here and now instead of waiting for someone to make a decision.

ORCID

Kanako Taku https://orcid.org/0000-0003-1515-7951

References

Horesh, D., & Brown, A. D. (2020). Traumatic stress in the age of COVID-19: A call to close critical gaps and adapt to new realities. *Psychological Trauma: Theory, Research, Practice and Policy*, *12*(4), 331–335. https://doi.org/10.1037/tra0000592

Johnston, C. S. (1995). The rokeach value survey: Underlying structure and multidimensional scaling. *The Journal of Psychology*, *129*(5), 583–597. https://doi.org/10.1080/00223980.1995.9914930

Kolyperas, D., Maglaras, G., & Sparks, L. (2019). Sport fans' roles in value co-creation. *European Sport Management Quarterly*, *19*(2), 201–220. https://doi.org/10.1080/16184742.2018.1505925

Warnke, K., & Paul, J. (2016). [Zika Virus – Impact on the 2016 Olympic Games in Rio de Janeiro]. *Sportverletzung Sportschaden: Organ der Gesellschaft fur Orthopadisch-Traumatologische Sportmedizin*, *30*(3), 154–156. https://doi.org/10.1055/s-0042-110251

Woratschek, H., Horbel, C., & Popp, B. (2014). The sport value framework: A new fundamental logic for analyses in sport management. *European Sport Management Quarterly*, *14*(1), 6–24. https://doi.org/10.1080/16184742.2013.865776

OPEN ACCESS

Defining a 'Risk Group' and Ageism in the Era of COVID-19

Atiqur Rahman and Yasmin Jahan

ABSTRACT

By classifying older adults, based on chronological age, as a higher risk group of coronavirus disease, 2019 is unacceptable and unfair- potentially reinforcing ageism. This ageist approach can accelerate the risk of social isolation, and heightened levels of psychosocial distress. Moreover, a general calculation of the number that is generated merely from the case fatality rate surely will mislead the indicators of the epidemic's trajectory, and lead to another *infodemic*. Therefore, transparency in news dissemination, the underlying health conditions and cultural differences of older adults are essential aspects while defining a risk group.

This paper puts forward a timely social issue that directs to the cumulative incidence of coronavirus disease (COVID-19), it addresses the classification of a higher risk group (infected and suspected older adults) by the outbreak which is not only questionable but also problematic.

Global responses to COVID-19 pandemic are in pace considering the mode of transmission, exponential spread, and case fatality rate. Nearly every nation will have to deal with the consequences of COVID-19 as it will leave hundreds of thousands, possibly millions of survivors with long term mental distress and trauma. A simple age threshold and higher susceptibility of a specific group such as older adults compared to other age groups have also been espoused negatively both in policies (CDC., 2020a) and scientific writings (Li et al., 2020). For example, the case-fatality rate for COVID-19 is reported as 3–5%, 4–11%, and 10–27% for the age group between 65–74, 75–84, and above 85 years respectively. In contrast, no intensive care unit admissions or deaths are reported among persons aged ≤19 years till 16 March 2020 (CDC., 2020b). Information like this is retaining older adults as a higher risk group in estimating mortality and morbidity during the COVID-19 pandemic across the globe. The consequence, on the one hand, is manifesting a widespread misperception about the global impact of the outbreak while on the other hand is placing older adults into a confined zone of social exclusion (Le Couteur et al., 2020). This way of attempting to deal with this virus situation will bring discriminatory attitudes and trauma together toward older adults.

The immediate consequences are not only fostering discourses of exclusion toward older adults but also accelerating the risk of social isolation, and heightened levels of psychosocial distress. Moreover, the simplification of the crisis by labeling older adults as "highly vulnerable group" and ignoring their cultural, social as well as contextual differences could significantly impact on the survivor's psychological and physical conditions after the outbreak. Such an ageist approach, by definition, is a process of— systematic stereotyping and discrimination against people based on age alone- called ageism (Butler, 1975) would be completely unacceptable and unfair. Importantly, chronological age is a very poor argument to determine an individual's usual state of health and resilience.

It is worthwhile to be informed about the potential risk groups of the virus to follow preventive measures properly; however, the negligence of differences and stereotypes of the group could be problematic. According to WHO guidelines, to be classified as a risk group you are "at increased risk of severe illness from any diseases" (Public Health Emergency (PHE), 2015). However, the underlying differences being at risk may depend on various characteristics. For instance, individual's physical conditions, the chances of being cured considering a timeline, and behaviors that affect the likelihood of developing a disease. Therefore, singling out a group of people based merely on chronological age irrespective of their associated health conditions cannot be a unanimous determinant. A justifiable explanation needs to be distinguishing "labeling," "discrimination" and "prioritization" while targeting older adults in order to describe the global scale of an infectious disease like COVID-19.

The case detection rate is changing daily, and new information comes out about the clinical course of the virus. Therefore, accurate calculation of the case fatality rate has also been challenged for its underestimation and overestimation (Rajgor et al., 2020). A simple count of the number of associated deaths or confirmed cases only with headline statistics can mislead indicators of the epidemic's trajectory. The power of these statistical metrics is absolute. We already see the impacts of media reporting that influence public sentiments toward the outbreak such as panic buying, food hoarding, and behaviors toward the risk groups including isolation from grandparents. Moreover, note that blind belief in information what we see or hear from social media and standalone content consumption tendencies could create another harmful *infodemic* (Cinelli et al., 2020). In other words, the information spreading out from a volume of (questionable) platforms should not be assumed conclusively. For the current crisis, we need to immediately identify recently originated rumors and respond to public perceptions, attitudes, and behaviors around the outbreak. To this end, an interactive real-time platform along with the epidemiological situation and social dynamics of the affected groups could be helpful to reduce community discrimination. The positive utilization of social media platforms, in addition, will enhance the control measures and mitigate the evolving spread of misinformation. To combat the severe implications of the pandemic, we need to combat the pandemic of social media panic.

Hence, an age alone categorization of older adults in media reporting will disproportionately impact mental health issues by developing a range of psychological distresses including persistent depression, stigmatization, psychotic symptoms, delirium, and even suicidality. However, there is currently very little known about COVID-19's broader impact on mental health problems and psychiatric symptoms of infected and suspected older adults. The post-outbreak psychosocial implications of COVID-19 can be overwhelming. There are good reasons to imagine the aftermath of mental stressors of the pandemic based on previous outbreaks experience such as severe acute respiratory syndrome (SARS) in 2003 (Xiang et al., 2020).

In short, we need more positive and supportive attitudes toward older adults from our living room to the electronic media sphere. The heterogeneity of underlying health conditions and social circumstances of older people are two important phenomenon needs to be acknowledged carefully. We suggest avoiding the chronological age alone perspective in presenting the global impact of COVID-19 which will otherwise reinforce and expedite ageism.

Acknowledgement

Both authors are thankful to Nadya Sotnychuk, Western Sydney University, Australia for her valuable comments.

Disclosure statement

No potential conflict of interest was reported by the author(s).

ORCID

Atiqur Rahman http://orcid.org/0000-0002-7675-2415
Yasmin Jahan http://orcid.org/0000-0001-9273-9651

References

Butler, R. N. (1975). Why survive? Being old in America. *Harper & Row*. Harper & Row.

CDC. (2020a). *People Who Are at Higher Risk for Severe Illness*. Retrieved from https://www.cdc.gov/coronavirus/2019-ncov/need-extra-precautions/people-at-higher-risk.html

CDC. (2020b). *Severe Outcomes Among Patients with Coronavirus Disease 2019 (COVID-19) —United States*. February 12–March 16, 2020. Retrieved from https://www.cdc.gov/mmwr/volumes/69/wr/mm6912e2.htm?s_cid=mm6912e2_w

Cinelli, M., Quattrociocchi, W., Galeazzi, A., Valensise, C. M., Brugnoli, E., Schmidt, A. L., & Scala, A. (2020). The covid-19 social media infodemic. arXiv Preprint arXiv, *2003.05004*.

Le Couteur, D. G., Anderson, R. M., & Newman, A. B. (2020). COVID-19 through the lens of gerontology. *The Journals of Gerontology: Series A, XX* (XX), 1–2. glaa080.https://doi.org/10.1093/gerona/glaa077

Li, Q., Guan, X., Wu, P., Wang, X., Zhou, L., Tong, Y., Ren, R., Leung, K. S. M., Lau, E. H. Y., Wong, J. Y., Xing, X., Xiang, N., Wu, Y., Li, C., Chen, Q., Li, D., Liu, T., Zhao, J., Liu, M., … Feng, Z. (2020). Early transmission dynamics in Wuhan, China, of novel coronavirus–infected pneumonia. *New England Journal of Medicine*, *382*(13), 1199–1207. https://doi.org/10.1056/NEJMoa2001316

Public Health Emergency (PHE). (2015). *Risk Groups*. Retrieved from https://www.phe.gov/s3/BioriskManagement/biosafety/Pages/Risk-Groups.aspx

Rajgor, D. D., Lee, M. H., Archuleta, S., Bagdasarian, N., & Quek, S. C. (2020). The many estimates of the COVID-19 case fatality rate. *The Lancet Infectious Diseases*.. https://doi.org/10.1016/S1473-3099(20)30244-9

Xiang, Y.-T., Yang, Y., Li, W., Zhang, L., Zhang, Q., Cheung, T., & Ng, C. H. (2020). Timely mental health care for the 2019 novel coronavirus outbreak is urgently needed. *The Lancet Psychiatry*, *7*(3), 228–229. https://doi.org/10.1016/S2215-0366(20)30046-8

Knowledge, Attitudes, Anxiety, and Coping Strategies of Students during COVID-19 Pandemic

Erick T. Baloran

ABSTRACT
COVID-19 is a global concern affecting Higher Education Institutions (HEIs). This pandemic led to a strong reaction among students who experiences anxiety. This cross-sectional study aimed to examine students' knowledge, attitudes, anxiety, and coping strategies during the COVID-19 pandemic. Results showed that students possessed sufficient knowledge and high-risk perceptions. Non-medical prevention measures were perceived as highly effective. Students were satisfied with the government's actions to mitigate problems. However, an unwillingness with the online-blended learning approach was observed. Students utilized various ways to cope up with mental health challenges. It is necessary to address students' mental health during this COVID-19 pandemic among HEIs.

Introduction

In January 2020, the WHO declared the outbreak of novel coronavirus infection, COVID-19, as a public health emergency of worldwide concern (World Health Organization, 2020a). The first recorded death outside Wuhan, China, was in the Philippines on February 20, 2020, and WHO declared COVID-19 in March 2020 as a pandemic (World Health Organization, 2020b). In the Philippines, WHO has been working with the Department of Health (DOH) and other national stakeholders and partners to increase the country's capability to address the COVID-19 pandemic (World Health Organization, 2020c). Besides, the DOH participated in the WHO Solidarity trial to assist in COVID-19 global response (World Health Organization, 2020d). Moreover, Enhanced Community Quarantine (ECQ) was implemented by the government to help the country's efforts to curb the adverse impacts of the COVID-19 pandemic (David et al., 2020). In the context of social impact, the COVID-19 crisis in the country appears that the effect is on the lower-income classes (National Economic and Development Authority, 2020).

Since the start of the COVID-19 pandemic, the psychological and emotional impact is also evident. Its emergence and spread create a lot of concern for people leading to increased levels of anxiety (Roy et al., 2020). COVID-19 crisis has also made an impact on the context of Philippine Education. Classes were postponed due to lockdown. The majority of colleges and universities also faced current challenges with virtual learning (Talidong & Toquero, 2020). In particular, Higher Education Institutions (HEIs) are prompted to establish management approaches regarding pandemics to encourage positive health behavior among students (Akan et al., 2010). Considering the relevance of all the above conditions, this study aimed to assess knowledge, attitudes, anxiety, and personal coping strategies of college students during the COVID-19 pandemic in Southern Philippines.

Methods

This was a cross-sectional study conducted among two local private colleges in the province of Davao del Sur, Southern Philippines, from April 25 – May 8, 2020. The researcher conducted this study during the increasing rate of COVID-19 pandemic cases in the Philippines, where Davao del Sur was under Enhanced Community Quarantine. Student respondents were determined using the snowball technique who answered the online survey developed through Google forms with an appended consent form. The survey link was sent to the student respondents via social media. The set of questions was adapted from the study of Akan et al. (2010), Khalid et al. (2016), and Roy et al. (2020) and was modified to suit in the context of the study. The study involved only those students who had access to the internet. There were a total of 530 students, including college and senior high school, who responded in the online survey.

Results and discussion

Among the 530 students who answered the questionnaire, 312 (58.87%) were female, 200 (37.73%) were male, and 18 (3.40%) were members of the LGBTQ + community. The majority of the students belong to the age group of 20 to 25-years-old (282 or 53.21%) and were single (502 or 94.72%), with below ten thousand Philippine peso monthly family income (350 or 66.04%). Moreover, the majority of the students' courses were in the field of law enforcement (121 or 22.83%).

In view of students' knowledge about COVID-19, a full 73.58% (390/530) of the students knew that the COVID-19 could spread through touching, sneezing, kissing, and food. They were aware that the primary symptom of the COVID-19 infection is fever (517/530 or 97.55%). Also, 91.70%

(486/530) of the students understood the importance of staying at home as a precautionary measure to stop the spread of the virus in the community. Previous studies provided evidence that COVID-19 is mainly transmitted through social contact with symptomatic persons (Burke et al., 2020; Chan et al., 2020; Huang et al., 2020; Li et al., 2020; Liu et al., 2020; Ong et al., 2020); with mild to severe symptoms (World Health Organization, 2020f), and through asymptomatic transmission (World Health Organization, 2020e). Besides, older persons (Kluge, 2020) and children (Dong et al., 2020; Lu et al., 2020) are at a considerably increased risk of serious illness after infection from COVID-19.

In terms of the perceptions of students on the risks of COVID-19 and the effectiveness of precautionary measures, 332/530 (62.64%) perceived a high-risk level of becoming infected. Also, students have seen the following as highly effective: social distancing and wearing a face mask (60%), hand washing and sanitizing (66.42%), and staying at home (84.72%). 74.15% (393/530) agreed on mass testing, and 90.19% (478/530) agreed with the implementation of Enhanced Community Quarantine (ECQ). Likewise, David et al. (2020) of the University of the Philippines emphasized that the implementation of the ECQ is effective in dropping the rate of transmission of the virus, which includes guidelines such as general physical distancing, mass testing and contact tracing, and strict home quarantine.

Given students' attitudes toward COVID-19 vaccination, the vast majority of student respondents (431/530 or 81.32%) stated that they were willing to be vaccinated against COVID-19, while only 18.68% (99/530) said they wouldn't be. Among those students who were unwilling to be vaccinated, 45.45% (45/99) said that it is not safe since it could have health risks or side effects. This is comparable to the findings of the study of Akan et al. (2010), which revealed that the main concerns of college students are related to the vaccination's safety during the pandemic influenza A/H1N1.

Moreover, 55.85% (296/530) had very high satisfaction with the services rendered by the local frontline workers, 41.51% (220/530) had very high satisfaction and confidence with the information dissemination done by the government, and 40.94% (217/530) were highly satisfied with the government's mitigations and actions to stop the spread of the virus. This is in parallel with the results of the study conducted by Hanrahan (2020), which exposed that seven in 10 Australians were generally satisfied with governments' actions in handling the COVID-19 pandemic.

Concerning the attitudes of students toward schooling during the COVID-19 pandemic, Table 1 showed that 80.38% (426/530) agreed with the stoppage of schools, and 65.85% (349) approved with the extension of the opening of classes for the next semester due to COVID-19 pandemic situation. However, 59.25% (314/530) disagreed with the conduct of the

Table 1. Students' attitudes toward schooling during COVID-19 pandemic ($n = 530$).

	Yes, *n* (%)	No, *n* (%)	I don't know, *n* (%)
Do you agree with the stoppage of schools during the COVID-19 pandemic?	426 (80.38)	37 (6.98)	67 (12.64)
Do you agree with the extension of the opening of classes for the next semester?	349 (65.85)	93 (17.55)	88 (16.60)
Do you agree with the conduct of the Online-Blended Learning Approach during the community quarantine?	169 (31.89)	314 (59.25)	47 (8.87)
The reasons for saying "YES" to Online-Blended Learning		*n* (%)	
a. I want to finish my academic requirements		136 (80.47)	
b. I don't want to quit school		92 (54.44)	
c. I am bored at home, and I miss doing academic tasks		48 (28.40)	
d. Online classes and modules are more convenient and practical than going to school		71 (42.01)	
e. It is about time to use online-blended education in college especially during a crisis like this		90 (53.25)	
f. It would be safe to study at home than to go to school		137 (81.07)	
Total		169 (100)	
The reasons for saying "NO" to Online-Blended Learning			
a. I don't have an internet connection		227 (72.29)	
b. I don't have personal computers and smartphones		124 (39.49)	
c. I find online class and modules challenging to do		130 (41.40)	
d. I would still prefer learning inside the classrooms		194 (61.78)	
e. I find online classes and modules boring		41 (13.06)	
f. I cannot learn through online class and modules		112 (35.67)	
g. I don't have a personal interaction with my teacher and classmates		84 (26.75)	
h. I don't have budget or finances for an online class and online submissions of requirements/tasks		179 (57.01)	
Total		314 (100)	

Online-Blended Learning Approach. The primary reason for these students was poor internet connection (227/314 or 72.29%). Besides, the study conducted by Ja'ashan (2015) revealed that the majority of students who undergone online-blended learning expressed negative impressions due to slow internet connectivity.

Additionally, the majority of the students displayed anxiety during the entire period of lockdown. 62.64% (332/530) were worried about food and financial resources, and about 54% to 56% of the students avoid social contact, large meetings, and gatherings (Table 2). This confirmed the research of Roy et al. (2020), which reported individuals were worried for themselves and their families during the on-going pandemic. People could have limited social contact and avoided mass meetings. Besides, Lee (2020) affirmed that the COVID-19 pandemic affects students' mental health.

For the ways to cope up with the anxiety during the COVID-19 pandemic, students responded common personal coping strategies, as shown in Table 3. 90.19% (478) followed strict personal protective measures and about 80% avoid going out in public places to reduce exposure from COVID-19. This is line with the study of various authors (Faye et al., 2015; Khalid et al., 2016) which revealed that during virus outbreak, it is crucial for individuals to follow very stringent infection control practices with standard precautions and minimized public exposure.

Table 2. Students' anxiety related to COVID-19 pandemic ($n = 530$).

For the last week		*n* (%)
1.	I often think about COVID-19 pandemic	269 (50.75)
2.	I often feel paranoid about contacting the novel Corona Virus infection	143 (26.98)
3.	I often avoid partying	234 (44.15)
4.	I usually avoid social contact	297 (56.04)
5.	I typically avoid large meetings and gatherings	287 (54.15)
6.	I usually avoid doing physical exercise outside the home	189 (35.66)
7.	I often avoid ordering food online	118 (22.26)
8.	I usually avoid buying food in public markets and foodservice establishments	178 (33.58)
9.	I usually have talked with friends about the corona pandemic	154 (29.06)
10.	I often had difficulty sleeping by being worried about the Corona Virus pandemic	98 (18.49)
11.	I often feel affected by the posts on social media about Corona Virus infection	176 (33.21)
12.	I often feel affected by the talks of novel Corona Virus pandemic on the newspaper and news channels	123 (23.21)
13.	I often feel the need to buy and stock all essentials at home	169 (31.89)
14.	I often get afraid if anyone in my social circle or friends reports of being sick	185 (34.91)
15.	I often feel the need to use the sanitizer/gloves	198 (37.36)
16.	I often feel the need to wash my hands constantly	243 (45.85)
17.	I often feel worried about myself and my family regarding the spread of COVID-19 Viral Infection	274 (51.70)
18.	I usually use a mask without any apparent signs and symptoms of the infection	199 (37.55)
19.	The Idea of Novel Corona Viral Infection often makes me nervous leading to inappropriate behaviors with anyone	101 (19.06)
20.	The Idea of Novel Corona Viral Infection often makes me nervous that leads me to post on social media	67 (12.64)
21.	I often consider anybody I encounter as positive of the virus	99 (18.68)
22.	I am usually worried about my studies because of the lockdown	256 (48.30)
23.	I am often concerned about our food and financial resources during the lockdown	332 (62.64)

Table 3. Students' personal coping strategies during COVID-19 pandemic ($n = 530$).

During the community quarantine		*n* (%)
1.	Follow strict personal protective measures (e.g., mask, handwashing, etc.)	478 (90.19)
2.	Read about COVID-19, its prevention and mechanism of transmission	365 (68.87)
3.	Avoid going out in public places to minimize exposure from COVID-19	426 (80.38)
4.	Do relaxation activities, for example, involved in meditation, sports, exercise, music, etc.	119 (22.45)
5.	Praying, worshiping and Bible study	207 (39.06)
6.	Chat with family and friends to relieve stress and obtain support	259 (48.87)
7.	Use social media and social networks such as Facebook, Twitter, Tiktok, Youtube, etc.	312 (58.87)
8.	Play online games and computer games	153 (28.87)
9.	Talk and motivate myself to face the COVID-19 outbreak with a positive attitude	154 (29.06)
10.	Get help from family physicians or other doctors to reduce my stress and get reassurance	63 (11.89)
11.	Try to be busy at home in activities that would keep my mind away from COVID-19	247 (46.60)
12.	Avoid media news about COVID-19 and related fatalities	80 (15.09)
13.	Vent emotions by crying, screaming, etc.	47 (8.87)

Conclusion and recommendations

The COVID-19 pandemic posed significant concerns among students, especially among communities in the Southern Philippines. Based on the findings of this study, the students were aware of the COVID-19 pandemic and possessed sufficient knowledge about this global concern even though there were still gaps in various points. Students understood how the virus is spread, its symptoms, and the precautionary measures needed to be done by both individuals and the general community. They also professed the need to conduct mass testing and maintain enhanced community quarantine in every local community. Considering WHO's recommendation, students abide by the idea toward the COVID-19 vaccine, although a considerable percentage of some students showed distrust. In the context of education, students were reluctant toward the implementation of online-blended learning approach due to technological and financial constraints. During this COVID-19 pandemic, students were responsive and satisfied with the government's initiatives to limit the spread of infection.

Though there was increased anxiety felt by students regarding getting the COVID-19 infection, there is still enough evidence that students among two local colleges in Southern Philippines practice measures to deal with anxiety during this threat of global health security. In the future, HEIs should strengthen its plans on management strategies concerning outbreaks and pandemics, which may affect local communities. HEIs should also develop an innovative and helpful approach to promote and address the mental health issues of students during a pandemic. More importantly, though the Philippines is still at the stage of embracing the paradigm shift in pedagogical delivery, schools should start training students and teachers on the application of online-blended learning approach and improve Information and Communication Technology (ICT) resources and capacities of both teachers and students. The government subsidy and educational support in the future should include capacitating Filipino learners in using online tools considering health challenges like this or other community emergencies during any future.

References

Akan, H., Gurol, Y., Izbirak, G., Ozdatli, S., Yilmaz, G., Vitrinel, A., & Hayran, O. (2010). Knowledge and attitudes of university students toward pandemic influenza: A cross-sectional study from Turkey. *BMC Public Health, 10*(1), 1–8. https://doi.org/10.1186/1471-2458-10-413

Burke, R. M., Midgley, C. M., Dratch, A., Fenstersheib, M., Haupt, T., & Holshue, M. (2020). Active monitoring of persons exposed to patients with confirmed COVID-19 —

United States, January–February 2020. *Morbidity and Mortality Weekly Report, 69*(9), 245–246. https://doi.org/10.15585/mmwr.mm6909e1externalicon.

Chan, J., Yuan, S., Kok, K., To, K. K.-W., Chu, H., Yang, J., Xing, F., Liu, J., Yip, C. C.-Y., Poon, R. W.-S., Tsoi, H.-W., Lo, S. K.-F., Chan, K.-H., Poon, V. K.-M., Chan, W.-M., Ip, J. D., Cai, J. P., Cheng, V. C. C., Chen, P. H., … Hui, C. K.-M. (2020). A familial cluster of pneumonia associated with the 2019 novel coronavirus indicating person-to-person transmission: A study of a family cluster. *The Lancet, 395*(10223), 514–523. https://doi.org/10.1016/S01406736(20)30154-9

David, G., Rye, R. S., Agbulos, M. A. (2020, April 22). *COVID-19 forecasts in the Philippines: Insights for policy making (Updated as of April 22, 2020).* UP Media and Public Relations Office. https://www.up.edu.ph/covid-19-forecasts-in-the-philippines-insights-for-policy-making-updated-as-of-april-22-2020/

Dong, Y., Mo, X., & Hu, Y. (2020). Epidemiological characteristics of 2143 pediatric patients with 2019 coronavirus disease in China. *Pediatrics.* Advance online publication. https://doi.org/10.1542/peds.2020-0702

Faye, O., Boelle, P. Y., Heleze, E., Faye, O., Loucoubar, C., Magassouba, N., Soropogui, B., Keita, S., Gakou, T., Bah el, H. I., Koivogui, L., Sall, A. A., & Cauchemez, S. (2015). Chains of transmission and control of Ebola virus disease in Conakry, Guinea, in 2014: An observational study. *The Lancet, 15*(3), 320–326. https://doi.org/10.1016/S1473-3099(14)71075-8

Hanrahan, C. (2020, April 16). Coronavirus response wins support — but we're less happy with other Aussies' behaviour. *ABC News.* https://www.abc.net.au/news/2020-04-16/coronavirus-numbers-government-support-survey-data/12147292

Huang, C., Wang, Y., Li, X., Ren, L., Zhao, J., Hu, Y., Zhang, L., Fan, G., Xu, J., Gu, X., Cheng, Z., Yu, T., Xia, J., Wei, Y., Wu, W., Xie, X., Yin, W., Li, H., Liu, M., … Cao, B. (2020). Clinical features of patients infected with 2019 novel coronavirus in Wuhan. *The Lancet, 395*(10223), 497–506. https://doi.org/10.1016/S0140-6736(20)30183-5

Ja'ashan, M. (2015). Perceptions and attitudes towards blended learning for English courses: A case study of students at University of Bisha Mohammed. *English Language Teaching, 8*(9), 40–50.

Khalid, I., Khalid, T., Qabajah, M., Barnard, A., & Qushmaq, I. (2016). Healthcare workers emotions, perceived stressors and coping strategies during a MERS-CoV outbreak. *Clinical Medicine & Research, 14*(1), 7–14. https://doi.org/10.3121/cmr.2016.1303

Kluge, H. H. (2020, April 2). *Statement - Older people are at highest risk from COVID-19, but all must act to prevent community spread.* World Health Organization. http://www.euro.who.int/en/health-topics/health-emergencies/coronavirus-covid-19/statements/statement-older-people-are-at-highest-risk-from-covid-19,-but-all-must-act-to-prevent-community-spread.

Lee, J. (2020). Mental health effects of school closures during COVID-19. *The Lancet.* Advance online publication. https://doi.org/10.1016/S2352-4642(20)30109-7

Li, Q., Guan, X., Wu, P., Wang, X., Zhou, L., Tong, Y., Ren, R., Leung, K. S. M., Lau, E. H. Y., Wong, J. Y., Xing, X., Xiang, N., Wu, Y., Li, C., Chen, Q., Li, D., Liu, T., Zhao, J., Liu, M., … Feng, Z. (2020). Early transmission dynamics in Wuhan, China, of novel coronavirus-infected pneumonia. *New England Journal of Medicine, 382*(13), 1199–1207. https://doi.org/10.1056/NEJMoa2001316

Liu, J., Liao, X., Qian, S., Yuan, J., Wang, F., Liu, Y., Wang, Z., Wang, F.-S., Liu, L., Zhang, Z. (2020). Community transmission of severe acute respiratory syndrome coronavirus 2, Shenzhen, China. *Emerging Infectious Diseases.* Advance online publication. Doi: doi.org/ https://doi.org/10.3201/eid2606.200239.

Lu, X., Zhang, L., Du, H., Zhang, J., Li, Y. Y., Qu, J., Zhang, W., Wang, Y., Bao, S., Li, Y., Wu, C., Liu, H., Liu, D., Shao, J., Peng, X., Yang, Y., Liu, Z., Xiang, Y., Zhang, F., … Wong, G. W. K. (2020). Chinese Pediatric Novel Coronavirus Study Team. SARS-CoV-2 infection in children. *The New England Journal of Medicine, 382*(17), 1663–1665. https://doi.org/10.1056/NEJMc2005073

National Economic and Development Authority. (2020, March 19). *Addressing the social and economic impact of the COVID-19 pandemic.* NEDA. http://www.neda.gov.ph/wp-content/uploads/2020/03/NEDA_Addressing-the-Social-and-Economic-Impact-of-the-COVID-19-Pandemic.pdf

Ong, S. W. X., Tan, Y. K., Chia, P. Y., Lee, T. H., Ng, O. T., Wong, M. S. Y., & Marimuthu, K. (2020). Air, surface environmental, and personal protective equipment contamination by severe acute respiratory syndrome coronavirus 2 (SARS-CoV-2) from a symptomatic patient. *JAMA, 323*(16), 1610. https://doi.org/10.1001/jama.2020.3227

Roy, D., Tripathy, S., Kar, S., Sharma, N., Verma, S., & Kaushal, V. (2020). Study of knowledge, attitude, anxiety & perceived mental healthcare need in Indian population during COVID-19 Pandemic. *Asian Journal of Psychiatry, 51*, 102083–102087. https://doi.org/10.1016/j.ajp.2020.102083

Talidong, K. J. B., & Toquero, C. M. D. (2020). Philippine teachers' practices to deal with anxiety amid COVID-19. *Journal of Loss and Trauma.* Advance online publication. https://doi.org/10.1080/15325024.2020.1759225

World Health Organization. (2020a, March 18). *Mental health and psychosocial considerations during the COVID-19 outbreak.* WHO. https://www.who.int/docs/default-source/coronaviruse/mental-health-considerations.pdf

World Health Organization. (2020b, May 13). *Rolling updates on coronavirus disease (COVID-19).* WHO. https://www.who.int/emergencies/diseases/novel-coronavirus-2019/events-as-they-happen

World Health Organization. (2020c, March 18). *WHO supports the Philippine government in COVID-19 response.* WHO. https://www.who.int/docs/default-source/coronaviruse/mental-health-considerations.pdf

World Health Organization. (2020d, April 22). PH *Solidarity trial for COVID-19 treatments receives green light from ethics review body.* WHO. https://www.who.int/philippines/news/detail/22-04-2020-ph-solidarity-trial-for-covid-19-treatments-receives-green-light-from-ethics-review-body

World Health Organization. (2020e, April 2). *Coronavirus disease 2019 (COVID-19) Situation Report – 73.* WHO. https://www.who.int/docs/default-source/coronaviruse/situation-reports/20200402-sitrep-73-covid-19.pdf?sfvrsn=5ae25bc7_2

World Health Organization. (2020f). *Coronavirus.* WHO. https://www.who.int/health-topics/coronavirus#tab=tab_3

Together for Hope and Resilience: A Humanistic Experience by the Vulnerability, Trauma, Resilience and Culture Lab Members during the COVID-19 Pandemic

Jude Mary Cénat, Pari-Gole Noorishad, Camille Blais-Rochette, Sara-Emilie McIntee, Joana N. Mukunzi, Wina Paul Darius, Cathy Broussard, Catherine Morse, Gloria Ukwu, Emmanuelle Auguste, and Kerry Menelas

ABSTRACT

The COVID-19 pandemic has brought stress and anxiety to students, professors, and staff in universities. The effectiveness of members of research laboratories not directly involved in research on the virus may be impacted. At the University of Ottawa, laboratories have been affected by the shutdown of all non-essential activities. An experience in a research laboratory at the University of Ottawa observed that members were affected by anxiety, stress, sleep deregulation, etc. However, a humanistic approach that allowed members to share their COVID-19 experiences in an authentic, empathic atmosphere leads them to regain their effectiveness, create hope, and develop resilience strategies.

With the progression of the COVID-19 pandemic, on March 13, 2020, the University of Ottawa announced the end of all non-essential activities on campus and the transition of all courses online as of March 18. In addition to the anxiety associated with the fear of being infected, these changes brought further stress to students, professors, and administrative staff in the different faculties of the University. The move to online courses raised many questions to which the University and its various faculties did not immediately have the appropriate answers to: How will courses be validated? What types of exams will be administered? How will online courses work? Given the limitations of current platforms, how will we be ready to launch online courses in less than a week? With provincial and federal governments announcing strict confinement measures, some students rushed home to their parents, with increasing stress, worry, and anxiety about the fear of being infected by the COVID-19 and the measures to prevent the spread of COVID-19 among local populations.

The COVID-19 pandemic and the effectiveness of the V-TRaC lab

This pandemic arrived at a particular time for the Vulnerability, Trauma, Resilience and Culture Laboratory (V-TRaC Lab) at the University of Ottawa because data collection for several projects was being launched during this period. Since the V-TRaC Lab works with vulnerable groups and communities, less conventional strategies are generally used by research assistants (usually students at the end of their undergraduate studies) to reach these populations. They go to churches, mosques, community organizations, student associations, community radio shows, cultural programs, sports teams, and youth associations to administer questionnaires, conduct interviews and focus groups, promote participation in data collection or educate and raise awareness on mental health issues or issues related to domestic violence. The confinement measures marked the end of a busy schedule that should have allowed the recruitment of participants for several projects, and social and community mobilization for others. However, some activities remained unaffected. For example, in the context of one of the Lab's projects, several systematic reviews with meta-analyses are being conducted simultaneously. Students (both research assistants and volunteers) involved in these projects have continued working from home with their research remaining unaffected by the events surrounding the COVID-19 pandemic. For other projects, new strategies have been put into place and should allow us to achieve at least half of our objectives in terms of recruitment and community mobilization. However, the days following the University of Ottawa's initiative to shut down non-essential services lead to a loss of efficiency among the members of the laboratory. Many teleconferences and mobilization meetings held with the members did not successfully allow our teams to catch their breaths and make progress on their respective projects. Losing many points of references at once is challenging and requires support in order to optimize adaptability (Cullen et al., 2014). This is where positive and authentic leadership plays an important role (Adams et al., 2019).

The establishment of a humanistic mutual support group

Initially wanting to check-in with his lab members, the director wrote to them, requesting an update on everyone's current situation. He also took the opportunity to launch a weekly teleconference meeting where the lab would share their objective and subjective experiences with the COVID-19 and specifically the confinement. Over the course of these meetings, a dynamic was established. A lot happened in the students' respective lives and many quickly adapted to their new reality. The students soon regained greater efficiency, which led to the implementation of new mobilization strategies, as well as the submission and publication of articles and an important psychological intervention guide meant for mental health professionals intervening in contexts of infectious disease epidemics (Cénat et al., 2020).

The one-and-a-half-hour group meetings were based on a rather integrative approach offering everyone the opportunity to share their experiences within a deeply caring, empathic, non-directive, non-judgmental, and humanistic group. The meetings were based on four main pillars:

- *Freedom to join as they please*: No lab member was forced to join the group call. However, as friendships and affinities developed at the V-TRaC Lab, students sometimes invited others to join the call and made it a habit to text and call each other for check-ins outside of the weekly meeting. The weekly meetings contributed to bring a renewed sense of purpose in this uncertain and unstable COVID-19 pandemic time, and to strengthen the sense of belonging among the lab members.
- *Discuss present pandemic-related experiences*: Discussions focused on the present lab members' experiences related to COVID-19. In addition to factual experiences, subjective concerns, fears, feelings, and emotions were also shared. Experiences of the "*here and now*" were discussed, building each person's capacity to elaborate. This technique made it possible for them to share their experiences within a caring and empathic group, and members often noticed that they were not alone in experiencing these emotions, fears, and worries.
- *Self-reflection and self-discovery, exploration of one's adaptability and resiliency during the pandemic*: The discussions also allowed the lab members to reflect on the adjustments they had had to make since the implementation of the confinement measures. Furthermore, techniques used to facilitate adaptation and resilience were shared. The confinement measures and the contagiousness of COVID-19 may lead some to develop behaviours that are observed in mental illnesses (e.g., obsessing about hand washing, panicking while grocery shopping, isolating from loved ones, etc.). At the end of the pandemic, it will be necessary to address inadaptive behaviors, and to adjust, and find the coping and resilience strategies needed to bounce back.
- *Offer respect and authenticity of expression in an egalitarian and non-directive sharing environment*: The meetings were conducted in a collaborative approach in order to encourage free, authentic, empathic, and non-directive speech. This allowed everyone to express themselves without fear of being judged or having to defend themselves. With respect and empathy, everyone was able to find their place, share their experiences, and grow, together, as a group.

Creativity and recovered efficiency

Instead of a formal discussion, we opted to analyze two main elements that emerged from this experience: the renewal of creative abilities and regained efficiency. Regarding the first element, in addition to sharing their experiences with confinement and the COVID-19 pandemic in words, members also began to share their artistic and culinary creations. As the meetings progressed, some members returned to cooking, some to painting, and some to writing poetry (see Image 1). As several studies have shown, resilience is above all a question of creativity (Cénat et al., 2015, 2019). Adapting requires creating a universe parallel to adversity in order to initiate a process of resilience. This is in fact what the lab members did. During our meetings, V-TRaC lab members read poetry, quotes, and texts, shared pictures of their paintings and home-cooked meals, and took new initiatives to help each other cope with the confinement measures and the time of uncertainty that the COVID-19 pandemic represents.

The second element that emerged in the group was that, over time, efficiency was recovered. In addition to the various projects that were relaunched, a positive energy emerged. This also enabled us to accelerate the pace at which we finalized a psychological intervention guide initially intended for low-and middle-income countries affected by Ebola virus disease. The guide was adapted to also address issues relating to COVID-19 and other epidemic contexts and was published in English and French (Cénat et al., 2020). This newfound efficiency was in part due to the group's empathy and humanistic approach used during the weekly support meetings. From the meetings, emerged a new dynamic, strong bonds, and the desire to work together. In the end, in conjunction with helping members develop resilience strategies, these meetings, which had no therapeutic focus, have promoted a sense of community that will outlive the pandemic. Knowing that others were experiencing similar difficulties and anxieties, similar emotions and concerns also made it possible to share strategies, to test them, to provide hope, and to engage in a collective process of resilience. In sum, checking in on others and sharing experiences helped people regain motivation in their personal and professional lives.

To conclude

This experience at the V-TRaC Lab showed that the COVID-19 pandemic reached different spheres of students' and researchers' lives. They were, like the majority of the population, affected by fear, worry, anxiety, exacerbation of stress, and sleep deregulation, among other consequences. It also showed that an approach based on caring, empathy, generosity, sharing of experiences, and humanism can help recover effectiveness and develop coping and resilience strategies. Often, resilience must be supported, and keeping research groups impersonal can result in losing bright students along the way. Researchers should not be afraid to develop such experiences because the trauma that cannot be symbolized is trauma that cannot be inscribed in the community of speaking beings (Cénat, 2018).

Disclosure statement

No potential conflict of interest was reported by the author(s).

References

Adams, B. G., Meyers, M. C., & Sekaja, L. (2019). Positive leadership: Relationships with employee inclusion, discrimination, and well-being. *Applied Psychology*, https://doi.org/10.1111/apps.12230

Cénat, J. M. (2018). *Traumas et résilience: lec¸ons du tremblement de terre de 2010 en Haïti*. Les Presses de l'Université Laval.

Cénat, J. M., Charles, C. H., & Kebedom, P. (2019). Multiple traumas, health problems and resilience among Haitian Asylum Seekers in Canada's 2017 migration crisis: Psychopathology of crossing. *Journal of Loss and Trauma*, 1–22. https://doi.org/10.1080/15325024.2019.1703610

Cénat, J. M., Derivois, D., Hébert, M., Eid, P., & Mouchenik, Y. (2015). Psychometric properties of the Haitian Creole version of the Resilience Scale with a sample of adult survivors of the 2010 earthquake. *Comprehensive Psychiatry*, *63*, 96–104. https://doi.org/10.1016/j.comppsych.2015.09.002

Cénat, J. M., McIntee, S. E., Noorishad, P.-G., Rousseau, C., Derivois, D., Birangui, J., Bukaka, J. Balayulu-Makila, O. (2020). *Psychological Intervention Guide: Intervene in the Context of Infectious Disease Outbreaks*. Ottawa: Niversité d'Ottawa, Université de Bourgogne Franche-Comté, McGill University, Université de Lubumbashi. https://app.mhpss.net/resource/guide-dintervention-psychologique-en-cas-depidemie-de-maladies-infectieuses

Cullen, K. L., Edwards, B. D., Casper, W. C., & Gue, K. R. (2014). Employees' Adaptability and Perceptions of Change-Related Uncertainty: Implications for Perceived Organizational Support, Job Satisfaction, and Performance. *Journal of Business and Psychology*, *29*(2), 269–280. https://doi.org/10.1007/s10869-013-9312-y

The Impact of Social Uncertainty, Protests, and COVID-19 on Hong Kong Teachers

Kevin M. Wong and Benjamin Luke Moorhouse

ABSTRACT
Teachers in Hong Kong endured an unprecedented 2019–2020 school year with widespread civil unrest followed by the COVID-19 pandemic. These events placed a great deal of stress on teachers as they navigated them with students in face-to-face and virtual environments. The current study examines how social uncertainty impacted ten primary and secondary school teachers in Hong Kong through semi-structured interviews. Findings indicated that the challenging events strengthened teacher motivation as they demonstrated greater commitment to teaching, a strong desire to journey with students through hardship, and a motivation to equip students with tools to navigate uncertain circumstances in the future.

"I haven't quite figured this out yet, but I do know that I've lost something."

– Luke, a secondary school teacher in Hong Kong

The 2019–2020 school year has been a period of uncertainty for education in Hong Kong. It started in September 2019 during widespread civil unrest triggered by the now suspended "2019 Hong Kong extradition bill," which led to temporary school closures, a number of adolescents arrested, and severe strain on relationships between sections of society (Purbrick, 2019) and the mental health of citizens (Hou & Hall, 2019). During this period, Hong Kong teachers were often placed in the difficult position of helping students make sense of the evolving situation while also receiving criticism and being called "instigators" for not doing enough to dissuade students from protesting (Sun et al. 2020). Then in February 2020, the COVID-19 pandemic forced schools to suspend face-to-face teaching and required teachers to provide alternative means to continue student learning (Chan, 2020). This required teachers to think of alternative instructional methods for learners while teaching and supporting students in different physical spaces (Moorhouse, 2020; Moorhouse & Beaumont, in press).

The impact of this period on teachers, and in particular on how they understand their role as teachers, has not been fully understood. On the one hand, the American Psychological Association (2020) acknowledged the potential trauma of social isolation due to COVID-19 on members of society, threatening feelings of loneliness, anxiety, depression and possible post-traumatic stress disorder. On the other hand, the Department of Mental Health at the World Health Organization (2020) noted that adults working with children should be mindful that children often observe adults' behaviors and emotions for cues on how to manage their own emotions. While teachers might need time and space to process and take care of their own well-being, they also inherently serve as role models for the children in their classrooms. In some circumstances, these juxtaposing messages may cause added stress on teachers, influencing their motivation to teach. Moreover, the pandemic "hit" during a period of extreme social tension and uncertainty caused by the Hong Kong protests, compounding the stress and anxiety of an already traumatized population (Purbrick, 2019).

Research indicates that teacher motivation is an essential component in effective classrooms (Han & Yin, 2016). Although teacher motivation derives primarily from an "intrinsic value of teaching" (Han & Yin, 2016, p. 7), it can be undermined by various factors, including stress and anxiety (Dörnyei & Ushioda, 2011), and ambiguous and conflicting role demands (Han & Yin, 2016). These factors are likely to be more pronounced during periods of social uncertainty, such as those caused by civil unrest, protests, or a pandemic (Kumar & Rajasekharan Nayer, 2020; Talidong & Toquero, 2020).

This small-scale exploratory study reports on part of a larger study that examined teachers' responses to the COVID-19 school suspensions. The current study specifically aimed to understand the impact of the social uncertainties evident in the 2019–2020 school year on teachers working in Hong Kong schools. More specifically, it sought to examine the experiences of teachers and how these social uncertainties have influenced their motivations to teach. The study was guided by the research question: How have the COVID-19 pandemic and the 2019 Hong Kong protests impacted teacher motivation?

By understanding this impact on teacher motivation, school administrators, government officials and teacher educators can become more aware of how to best support the needs of teachers on the frontline during periods of social unrest.

Methods

Participants included primary ($N = 5$) and secondary ($N = 5$) school teachers working in Hong Kong schools. Novice and experienced teachers working in all three main regions of Hong Kong were represented. The sample included seven female and three male teachers, reflecting the gender ratio of the teaching profession in Hong Kong. Through convenience sampling, teachers first completed a survey as part of a larger study in March 2020. Findings from the survey informed the development of the interview guide for the current study. Participants engaged in individual semi-structured interviews lasting 55–70 minutes conducted over video conferencing software to minimize human-to-human contact in April 2020. All participants were informed of their rights and provided informed consent. Interviews were audio-recorded to facilitate the transcription process for data analysis. Interviews are a common data collection method that help researchers see knowledge as "generated between humans, often through conversation" (Cohen et al., 2011). They also allow researchers to dig deeper into participants' perceptions and experiences (Cohen et al., 2011). Interviews are an appropriate method to use during changing and unpredictable events (e.g., during civil unrest or a pandemic) as they help researchers understand the lived experiences of those affected. In this study, participants are referred to by pseudonyms to protect their identities.

Data were analyzed using thematic analysis with the six-stage process proposed by Braun and Clarke (2006). Themes were identified, enumerated, analyzed and reported with rich descriptions of data (Braun & Clarke, 2006). Throughout the process, the researchers kept in communication and discussed differences in interpretations. Two salient themes emerged from the analysis.

Findings

The impact of social uncertainty on teachers' commitments

In Hong Kong, the 2019–2020 school year has been dominated by protests and the COVID-19 pandemic, leading to widespread social uncertainty (Purbrick, 2019). Yet these experiences appeared to solidify educators' commitment to the teaching profession and enhance intrinsic motivation to teach.

When the teachers were asked to reflect upon the effects of these events on their motivation, their concern for students' mental and physical well-being was the most salient theme. For example, when discussing the impact of the pandemic, David noted, "Some of my students have parents who are doctors … they would suddenly break down and just tell [me] something's wrong, something's wrong, something's wrong." Meanwhile, Flora worried about the safety of her students during the protests as "radicals" were "on the streets … damaging everything!"

Teachers were worried about their students. They understood that events of the school year had taken a toll on students' well-being and indicated that the repercussions of social unrest would "impact" students "for the long run." In response, teachers shared that they had to shift their role as educators to strongly consider their students "not just as learners, but as people." Indeed, Luke shared that he would take his time to logout of virtual class meetings because there would often be one or two students who were slow to log off and wanted somebody to talk to. Kitty shared about a conversation with a student who was considering suicide because she missed human interaction. Without question, teachers were motivated to be present for students.

In fact, teachers commented on how they were able to uniquely empathize with students who were also caught in the middle of protests and school closures. This meant teachers had to reconsider their roles in the classroom as they personally navigated and simultaneously helped students navigate the unprecedented circumstances. Medina noted, "It really feels like I'm going through all of this with them." She shared that she needed to consider "the different sides of being a teacher" to best support her students. Educators appeared motivated to not only be present for students, but committed to journeying with them through times of uncertainty.

Journeying with students, however, presented an interesting tension as certain teachers had to discern whether or not politics belonged in the classroom. On the one hand, teachers wanted to share their convictions with students to help them make sense of all the uncertainty before them. On the other hand, teachers felt the need to maintain a sense of professionalism, which meant staying politically neutral in the classroom. Kitty shared the tension she felt,

> It's really hard to express our ideas … based on facts, so we are puzzled about what the [facts are] … and how to convey the message to the students. [At] school we need to be politically neutral but it's really hard because we also have our personal opinion but we don't express our personal opinion in front of students.

Still, Kitty resolved that if she, as a teacher, still had power to influence her students and guide them toward the truth, she wanted to "finish the job until the end."

The impact of social uncertainty on pedagogy and instruction

In this time of social unrest, educators noted the importance of adapting their instruction to cultivate critical thinking skills so students could discern facts from opinions when seeking truth. The 2019 protests led to polarizing media coverage with extreme views from either "yellow" (pro-democracy) or "blue" (pro-establishment) camps. Charis said, "I had students who didn't really have a good understanding of what the protest was for, but they just randomly chanted things [during class] … As educators, we need to really help students … learn how to think critically."

Relatedly, Charis shared her motivation to cultivate conversations in class on critical issues. She recalled an instance when her students did not treat her Korean colleague well because COVID-19 had recently ravaged the nation of South Korea. Although her colleague had not returned to South Korea, students were making assumptions without any justification. "It's things like this where you … hope they can develop to become … kind-hearted people who treat everybody equally," Charis noted. "I think these outside societal events kind of help shape [students' perspectives]" and can serve as another learning opportunity.

As events continued to unfurl in the 2019–2020 academic year, educators were motivated to use societal events to engage students in learning in meaningful and relevant ways. The following excerpt from Luke illustrates this motivation,

> This is also an amazing opportunity to make what you're teaching in the classroom relevant and alive for students. I mean I'm lucky that I'm a teacher. When we were … studying China and authoritarian regimes, and the protests happened, … I don't need to sell or convince my students that what we're learning is relevant to their lives. It is!

Likewise, Madina shared how read-alouds from Shel Silverstein and The Giving Tree allowed her to make real-life connections and applications about how to love people in society during civil unrest and consider the needs of family members when at home during a pandemic.

Discussion and Conclusion

This small-scale study explored how social uncertainties caused by the COVID-19 pandemic and the 2019 Hong Kong protests impacted teachers and their motivation to teach. Findings suggest that the unique experiences of the 2019–2020 school year strengthened teacher motivation and the intrinsic value that teaching affords them (Han & Yin, 2016). More specifically, teachers have a greater commitment to teaching and a desire to journey with their students as they face social uncertainties together. This commitment can help increase teachers' resilience during periods of uncertainty (Beltman et al., 2011) while placing them in a good position to support younger members of society as they try to make sense of traumatic experiences impacting them.

Teachers are aware of this role. They adjust their pedagogy and instruction to reflect the needs that arise from volatile situations, while conceptualizing their role beyond subject-content delivery to the development of the whole-learner, with specific emphasis on helping learners think critically. It is important that teachers are given autonomy to adapt content and instruction to prioritize student well-being over academic performance (Pearson & Moomaw, 2005).

Although the study has yielded valuable findings regarding teacher motivation during this period of social uncertainty, it is limited in scale and methods. Despite the urgency of examining teacher experiences in the current study, future research may consider larger longitudinal designs that use a variety of research methods to explore the perspectives and experiences of teachers in various contexts impacted by civil unrest, health emergencies, and other social stressors. This will help document some of the longer-term or lingering effects of social unrest on the teaching profession.

If social uncertainty continues for an extended period, the teachers' concerns for their students' mental and physical well-being may take a toll on their own mental health and long-term commitment to the profession (Dörnyei & Ushioda, 2011), which in turn can negatively affect student well-being (Han & Yin, 2016). While findings from this study suggest that teacher motivation is strengthened during challenging times, extended periods of social isolation or social unrest can lead to compounded, comorbid feelings of fear, anxiety, depression, anger, or stigmatization (APA, 2020). It is, therefore, important for school administrators, government officials and teacher educators to be mindful of the roles teachers adopt during such events, and to explore responsive ways of supporting teachers. For example, leaders may provide counseling and coping strategy training (Cole et al., 2013) to teachers as they navigate the complexities inherent within social unrest and unprecedented events with their students.

ORCID

Kevin M. Wong http://orcid.org/0000-0001-6237-0427
Benjamin Luke Moorhouse http://orcid.org/0000-0002-3913-5194

References

American Psychological Association (APA). (2020). Available from: https://www.apa.org/practice/programs/dmhi/research-information/social-distancing

Beltman, S., Mansfield, C., & Price, A. (2011). Thriving not just surviving: A review of research on teacher resilience. *Educational Research Review*, *6*(3), 185–207. https://doi.org/10.1016/j.edurev.2011.09.001

Braun, V., & Clarke, V. (2006). Using thematic analysis in psychology. *Qualitative Research in Psychology*, *3*(2), 77–101. https://doi.org/10.1191/1478088706qp063oa

Chan, H.-H. (16 March, (2020). Coronavirus: Hong Kong students adapt to online learning amid class suspension over pandemic. SCMP Online. Available from: https://www.scmp.com/news/hong-kong/education/article/3075280/coronavirus-hong-kong-students-adapt-online-learning-amid

Cohen, L., Manion, L., & Morrison, K. (2011). *Research methods in education* (7th ed.). Routledge.

Cole, R., Hayes, B., Jones, D., & Shah, S. (2013). Coping strategies used by school staff after a crisis: A research note. *Journal of Loss & Trauma*, *18*(5), 472–481. https://doi.org/10.1080/15325024.2012.719335

Dörnyei, Z., & Ushioda, E. (2011). *Teaching and researching motivation* (2nd ed.). Longman.

Han, J., & Yin, H. (2016). Teacher motivation: Definition, research development and implications for teachers. *Cogent Education*, *3*(1), 1217819. https://doi.org/10.1080/2331186X.2016.1217819

Hou, W. K., & Hall, B. J. (2019). The mental health impact of the pro-democracy movement in Hong Kong. *The Lancet Psychiatry*, *6*(12), 982. https://doi.org/10.1016/S2215-0366(19)30382-7

Kumar, A., & Rajasekharan Nayar, K. (2020). COVID 19 and its mental health consequences. *Journal of Mental Health*. https://doi.org/10.1080/09638237.2020.1757052

Moorhouse, B. L. (2020). Adaptations to a face-to-face initial teacher education course 'forced' online due to the COVID-19 pandemic. *Journal of Education for Teaching*, 1–3. DOI: https://doi.org/10.1080/02607476.2020.1755205

Moorhouse, B. L., & Beaumont, A. (in press). Utilizing video conferencing software to teach young language learners during face-to-face class suspensions caused by the COVID-19 pandemic. *TESOL Journal*.

Pearson, L. C., & Moomaw, W. (2005). The relationship between teacher autonomy and stress, work satisfaction, empowerment, and professionalism. *Educational Research Quarterly*, *29*(1), 38–54.

Purbrick, M. (2019). A report of the 2019 Hong Kong protests. *Asian Affairs*, *50*(4), 465–487. DOI: https://doi.org/10.1080/03068374.2019.1672397

Sun, F., Chiu, P., & Tsang, D. (2020, October 12). Hong Kong teachers in the firing line over surge in students joining anti-government protests, getting arrested. SCMP Online. Available from: https://www.scmp.com/news/hong-kong/politics/article/3032589/hong-kong-teachers-firing-line-over-surge-students-joining

Talidong, K. J. B., & Toquero, C. M. D. (2020). Philippine teachers' practices to deal with anxiety amid COVID-19. *Journal of Loss and Trauma*. DOI: https://doi.org/10.1080/15325024.2020.1759225

World Health Organization. (2020, March 18). Mental health and psychosocial considerations during the COVID-19 outbreak. https://www.who.int/docs/default-source/coronaviruse/mental-health-considerations.pdf

The Effects of Incriminating COVID-19 News on the Returning Indonesians' Anxiety

Mahir Pradana, Syahputra Syahputra, Aditya Wardhana, Budi Rustandi Kartawinata, and Candra Wijayangka

ABSTRACT
The World Health Organization (WHO) has declared the novel coronavirus (COVID-19) as a global pandemic. Governments have urged their citizens to return to their home countries. In the case of Indonesia, some new coverage about COVID-19 which is disseminated by major national media channels has negatively influenced Indonesian travelers' mental condition. Returning Indonesians face anxiety for having been labeled as "virus carriers." This article explores how sensationalism in media reports may affect society's perspective toward returning Indonesian tourists during the COVID-19 pandemic.

Introduction

On 11 March 2020, the WHO officially declared novelcoronavirus (COVID-19) as a pandemic (World Health Organization (WHO), 2020). The first recorded case in Indonesia was on 2 March 2020, when two Indonesians were infected after having contacts with several Japanese nationals (Ratcliffe, 2020). By 9 April 2020, cases of COVID-19 were detected in all provinces in Indonesia (CNN Indonesia, 2020). By 4 May 2020, Indonesia has recorded 11,587 cases of COVID-19 (CNN Indonesia, 2020a).

Since the first case was discovered within their territory, the Indonesian government has limited the visit of foreign nationals and advised its citizens abroad to return home. Therefore, a massive number of traveling Indonesians reentered Indonesian border in March and April 2020. However, a new concern emerged among the returning Indonesians. Several news reports in the media with incriminating tendencies have driven people to believe that aside of visiting foreigners, Indonesian returning travelers are seen as the culprits who bring COVID-19 home.

This article follows the works of Wen et al. (2020) and Zheng et al. (2020), which discussed how misleading reports and sensational coverage of COVID-19 caused discrimination against Chinese individuals. In the same direction, we see that prejudice against returning Indonesians have emerged because of misleading media reports. This condition predominantly affects their mental health, next to the concern of getting exposed to the pandemic. Therefore, this article provides insights from Indonesia, as well as joins the works of Wen et al. (2020) and Zheng et al. (2020) as encouragement for related research efforts on travelers' mental health in times of global health crisis.

Media coverage on returning Indonesian travelers

Since the second week of March 2020, the ministry of foreign affairs of Indonesia has urged Indonesian citizens overseas to come home. Indonesians who possess residence permits of other countries are advised to stay where they reside, but those who do not, especially tourists, are urged to return (Yasmin, 2020).

After arriving on Indonesian soil, they must do a self-quarantine for 14 days. According to Johns Hopkins University & Medicine (2020), people who have been exposed and who are at risk of COVID-19 are advised to practice self-quarantine. Two weeks is enough to know whether they turn sick and may infect others. In addition to monitoring if symptoms develop, being in quarantine means someone who might be exposed will not transmit the disease to others, assumingly they stay at home for a minimum of 14 days.

Self-quarantine and social distancing are two Indonesian government's main approach to prevent the contagion of COVID-19. Social distancing, which soon escalated to physical distancing, is principally the state of avoiding, attending or becoming part of large crowds. Citizens are also required to keep a distance from other people about 2 meters (Red Cross, 2020).

Theoretically, along with the urgency to wear masks in public places, these two essential activities are enough to prevent contagion (Talidong & Toquero, 2020). However, the fear spread by the media is inevitable. Due to the rising number of COVID-related deaths, Indonesian citizens began to fear visitors, regardless of their nationalities.

We conducted a small survey to see whether the returning Indonesians have done such preventive measures to combat COVID 19. We sent online questions to 40 faculty members at our university who returned from holiday and business trips in South Korea, India, Singapore and Malaysia within the period of February to April, 2020. The result showed that 40%

of them decided to self-quarantine at home and avoid crowded places, 36% of them decided to wear face masks everywhere they went, including when they only stayed at home, the rest of them suggested to wash hands regularly, exercise routinely and sleep longer. Around 99% believed that social distancing is effective as a preventive measure to prevent COVID-19.

Afterwards, we distributed different set of questions to their spouses, parents, children and neighbors to see whether they felt unsafe around the returning travelers. From 50 respondents, 95.4% agreed that they worried they might get infected or catch COVID-19 symptoms. This fear might also be related to the lack of government monitoring toward foreign visitors and returning Indonesians in February and March 2020. Several regions in Indonesia were also considered late in reinforcing self-quarantine and social distancing policy. People began to see returning Indonesians as virus carriers.

By the second week of April 2020, COVID-19 has infected over 4,000 citizens and caused 400 deaths in the country. News coverage plays a great role in triggering public anxiety and panic in the time of the COVID-19 pandemic. In these conditions, people can experience stress, fear, anxiety, and even anger (Wen et al., 2020). The urge to stay at home makes them only follow the news from newspapers, television and internet. Therefore, bombastic headlines such as "Dreadful! There Are More Than 300 Indonesian Citizens Overseas Infected by Corona!" will only raise prejudice against Indonesians who are about to return home (Syahrianto, 2020).

Expected roles of the media during the pandemic

Aside from policy regulating returning Indonesian tourists, the Indonesian Ministry of Foreign Affairs also issued an additional policy for foreign travelers related to COVID-19. The one month visit visa-free, Visa on Arrival (VOA), and free diplomatic or official visas are all postponed until further notice (Akhlas & Iswara, 2020). The media should play a bigger role in delivering this news to Indonesian society to prevent preconceived ideas about returning Indonesians or foreign citizens who decide to stay in Indonesia during the pandemic.

We believe that since mass media have played a role in affecting people's perception toward visitors to Indonesian soil, the media should not participate in causing excessive syndrome amid the stretching of the war against COVID-19. Media should play a more central role in neutralizing their tone of COVID-19-related news so that people face the present situation without fear (Zheng et al., 2020). We asked a question to our returning Indonesian respondents about whether they worried they might carry COVID-19 to their home environment, 99% of them responded "yes.' They all felt such anxiety after reading information about COVID-19 on the media.

According to communication media data from the Indonesian Ministry of Communication and Information Technology (2020), there are 2,011 registered online sites, 674 radio stations, 523 TV stations, and 567 publishers newspapers and magazines all over Indonesia. These media should work together with the government in a better direction of news coverage. The Ministry of Communication and Information has been in coordination with the National Disaster Management Agency and the Ministry of Health. Therefore, any new information and developments about COVID-19 should flow to the media from these doors to avoid public confusion.

Shared knowledge does not always mean the truth, so information producers should pay attention to any narrative they publish to the public (Gilchrist, 2018). Aside from the urgency of being accurate, any COVID-19-related news must be objective and fair. There is nothing more effective than mass media in building opinions and affecting public perspectives.

Conclusion

Biased and incriminating news connecting COVID-19 and returning Indonesians are detrimental to the harmony of Indonesian society as a whole. Indonesians who return from abroad tend to face prejudice and unpleasant treatment. As a result, these returning citizens may experience anxiety next to the risk of getting infected by the virus. This unwanted situation is unnecessary since the Indonesian government has already been socializing self-quarantine and social distancing policy for returning Indonesians.

This article urges the media offices to embrace the need for more responsible ways of doing business. They should provide non-incriminating news reports when informing the effects of COVID-19 to Indonesians abroad, especially the ones who decide to return to their home country. It is better to reduce and avoid sensational headlines and focus on factual information. Indonesian media are also required to keep updates from the Ministry of Communication and Information, Ministry of Health, and the National Disaster Management Agency to deliver factual and useful COVID-19—related news to the public.

Future empirical studies are encouraged to explore the effect of incriminating news toward returning Indonesians on their mental health. In the same vein, an investigation can also focus on how effective Indonesian media socialize the government's COVID-19 social policy.

Disclosure statement

No potential conflict of interest was reported by the author(s).

ORCID

Mahir Pradana http://orcid.org/0000-0003-4761-2891
Syahputra Syahputra http://orcid.org/0000-0001-8133-3648
Aditya Wardhana http://orcid.org/0000-0002-3732-9454
Budi Rustandi Kartawinata http://orcid.org/0000-0002-4670-1019
Candra Wijayangka http://orcid.org/0000-0003-0829-3189

References

Akhlas, A. W., Iswara, M. A. (2020). Virus spread starts to hit Indonesian tourism as foreign arrivals cool. *The Jakarta Post*. https://www.thejakartapost.com/news/2020/03/02/virus-spread-starts-to-hit-indonesian-tourism-as-foreign-arrivals-cool.html

CNN Indonesia. (2020a). *Corona update May 4: 11,587 positive, 1,954 cured*. https://www.cnnindonesia.com/nasional/20200504122422-20-499762/update-corona-4-mei-11587-positif-1954-orang-sembuh

CNN Indonesia. (2020b). *Corona virus: millions of Indonesian citizens will return to their homeland, the government is urged to quarantine them*. https://www.cnnindonesia.com/nasional/20200504122422-20-499762/update-corona-4-mei-11587-positif-1954-orang-sembuh

CNN Indonesia. (2020c). *Government: 72,351 people examined through corona PCR test*. https://www.cnnindonesia.com/nasional/20200430173426-20-499034/pemerintah-72351-orang-sudah-diperiksa-lewat-tes-pcr-corona

Gilchrist, A. D. (2018). Post-truth: An outline review of the issues and what is being done to combat it. *Ibersid: revista de Sistemas de Información y Documentación*, *12*(2), 13–24.

Indonesian Ministry of Communication and Information Technology. (2020). Direktorat Jenderal Informasi dan Komunikasi Publik. https://kominfo.go.id/content/detail/5707/direktorat-jenderal-informasi-dan-komunikasi-publik/0/unit_kerja

Johns Hopkins University & Medicine. 2020. Johns Hopkins COVID-19 Testing Insights Initiative. https://coronavirus.jhu.edu/

Ratcliffe, R. (2020). *First coronavirus cases confirmed in Indonesia amid fears nation is ill-prepared for outbreak.* https://www.theguardian.com/world/2020/mar/02/first-coronavirus-cases-confirmed-in-indonesia-amid-fears-nation-is-ill-prepared-for-outbreak

Red Cross. (2020). *Coronavirus – what social distancing means.* https://www.redcross.org/about-us/news-and-events/news/2020/coronavirus-what-social-distancing-means.html

Syahrianto, M. (2020). Parah, Total Ada Lebih dari 300 WNI di Luar Negeri Terinfeksi Corona [Dreadful! There are more than 300 Indonesian citizens overseas infected by corona]. *Warta Ekonomi.* https://www.wartaekonomi.co.id/read280777/parah-total-ada-lebih-dari-300-wni-di-luar-negeri-terinfeksi-corona

Talidong, K. J. B., & Toquero, C. M. D. (2020). Philippine teachers' practices to deal with anxiety amid COVID-19. *Journal of Loss and Trauma*, May 20 (In Press), 1–7. https://doi.org/10.1080/15325024.2020.1759225

Wen, J., Aston, J., Liu, X., & Ying, T. (2020). Effects of misleading media coverage on public health crisis: A case of the 2019 novel coronavirus outbreak in China. *Anatolia*, *31*(2), 331–336. https://doi.org/10.1080/13032917.2020.1730621.

World Health Organization. (2020). *Novel coronavirus (2019-nCoV): Situation report – 8.* https://www.who.int/docs/default-source/coronaviruse/situation-reports/20200128-sitrep-8-ncov-cleared.pdf

Yasmin, N. (2020a). Foreign ministry orders Indonesian travelers to return home as 48 test positive for Covid-19. *The Jakarta Globe.* https://jakartaglobe.id/news/foreign-ministry-orders-indonesian-travelers-to-return-home-as-48-test-positive-for-covid19.

Yasmin, N. (2020b). *More Indonesians abroad contract Covid-19 as countries extend travel bans.* https://jakartaglobe.id/news/more-indonesians-abroad-contract-covid19-as-countries-extend-travel-bans.

Zheng, Y., Goh, E., & Wen, J. (2020). The effects of misleading media reports about COVID-19 on Chinese tourists' mental health: a perspective article. *Anatolia: An International Journal of Tourism and Hospitality Research*, *31*(2), 337–334. https://doi.org/10.1080/13032917.2020.1747208.

COVID-19: An Australian Perspective

Jane Shakespeare-Finch, Holly Bowen-Salter, Miranda Cashin, Amalia Badawi, Ruth Wells, Simon Rosenbaum, and Zachary Steel

ABSTRACT
Australia looks to be one of those lucky countries that adopted an early public health response limiting community transmission of COVID-19 and avoiding the levels of acute hospitalization and fatality seen in other settings. Yet the pandemic came on the back of the largest bushfire season the country had seen which itself followed a sequence of climatic disasters involving drought, cyclones and floods. The social and economic impact of the COVID-19 response has been substantial with widespread loss of employment, social dislocation and health fears sparked across the nation. Findings from risk modeling and population surveillance provide preliminary evidence of increased burden of psychological distress, morbidity and risk of suicide resulting from the current crisis. We also highlight the mental health risk that may arise from increased sedentary behavior with the introduction of lockdown and physical distancing measures. We also outline the potently valuable role of drawing on salutogenic models including resilience and posttraumatic growth research for individual and broader community level need.

Following years of drought, in June of 2019 the bushfire season started extremely early in the northern part of Australia. Mostly uncontrolled, the fires made their way down the country reaching their peak in December 2019 and January 2020. By this time the fires had moved predominantly to the south east of the continent. The fires burned out-of-control devastating every natural and manmade obstacle in the path. More than a billion animals, 46 million acres of land, and nearly 6000 buildings were destroyed (Centre for Disaster Philanthropy, 2020; Dickman, 2020). Despite the enormity of the natural disaster with thousands of homes and buildings destroyed the immediate death toll managed to be restricted to 34 people, including volunteer and professional fire fighters (Centre for Disaster Philanthropy, 2020). In terms of affected areas, this was the largest fire front the country had faced in living memory and it was simply terrifying. Capital cities along the eastern States of the country were shrouded in smoke at extremely hazardous levels which made breathing difficult for many with modeling estimating 417 fatalities and an additional 4456 acute hospital presentations due to respiratory and cardiovascular complications (Borchers Arriagada et al., 2020). It was the towns, rural properties, and people that bore the brunt of the infernos. The large urban populations could do little but look on, relatively helpless, as people affected by the fires fled from their homes and gathered on the beaches or wherever they felt they had the best chance of survival. The nation and the world watched on as fire trucks surrounded by flames tipped over with the force of the fire and thick smoke left police, paramedics, volunteers and professional fire-fighters with little vision. Eventually, the fires came under control, as the rain began in mid-February. Then it rained, and it rained. Images from NASA (2020) show areas razed by the fire that became flood plains. Concurrently, Cyclone Uesi passed by the Queensland and New South Wales coastline, bringing damaging winds, more rain, and flash flooding.

At the height of the bushfires and floods, COVID-19 was taking hold in China, a country we have very close ties with. According to Cranston of the Financial Review (2019), Australia conducts nearly 40% of its trade with China. As the floodwaters receded, the virus was spreading at a rapid rate around the world. Countries responded differently, some with swift closure of borders such as Denmark and New Zealand, and others more slowly, like the UK and the USA. The World Health Organization (WHO) declared a pandemic on the 11th of March, 2020. Increasingly, most people in the world recognized this was an experience few had faced before and there was a need for immediate action to reduce infection, disease and deaths. Locking down was the order of the day for most countries and Australia was an early adopter of this strategy, albeit with errors along the way. The Federal Government started to close national borders in mid-March (Murphy & Karp, 2020). With new restrictions of movement being implemented on a rolling basis, everything changed for most people and for many that was, and continues to be, accompanied by fear, uncertainty, anxiety, and for others, apathy and denial. Work, school, parenting, business, security, relationships, friends, family, finances … it all changed and is still changing as we write this.

It is clear that the mental health situation for Australia is unlikely to involve massive trauma exposure for families and risk of PTSD due to effectiveness of the public health measures. However the numerous large-scale stressful events including the disruption caused by the COVID-19 public health measures is likely to lead to complex adjustment challenges, reactions and disorder (Steel, 2020). The International Classification of Diseases 11th Revision (World Health Organization, 2018) characterizes adjustment disorder by maladaptive levels of worry, rumination, and failures in adaptation that significantly impair important life domains. As we move through this era of COVID-19, we are in a position of needing to deal with myriad biopsychosocial stressors while still being in a new and unfolding situation.

A key differentiator of COVID-19 from the catastrophic stressors such as the bushfires and floods is the simultaneous and direct impact of its effect on all citizens nationally and globally. Even at the height of the 2019–2020 bushfires, a large number of community sectors were not directly affected by the fires and were, therefore, able to assist, whether that be as a volunteer or contributing to fundraising. In contrast, the proliferation of the virus has placed unprecedented demand on all people. The challenges arising from this global pandemic have placed a great demand on the psychosocial functioning of the population in multiple ways within Australia.

The few population indicators that are available in Australia suggest an immediate and substantial impact on the mental health and wellbeing of the population. The Australian government statistics agency (Australian Bureau of Statistics, 2020) has been collecting fortnightly COVID-19 impact survey data involving a representative sample of 1028 adults across Australia. Findings indicate 68% of those surveyed have been concerned or very concerned about their health due to the spread of COVID-19. Twice as many adults reported experiencing anxiety, nervousness and restlessness compared to pre-COVID-19 surveillance data and 1 in 5 reported (22%) high levels of loneliness. Rates of people reporting severe depression increased from 5% to 10%. Indicators from other data sources converge to suggest a widespread impact with the national mental health helpline (Lifeline, 2020) reporting a sustained 25% increase in calls since the pandemic onset and the National Kids Helpline reporting similar increases. Research conducted during past pandemics has demonstrated that anxiety can be helpful when it is positively associated with helpful behaviors such as hand washing and sanitizing (Wheaton et al., 2012). However, excessive fear, worry and anxiety are likely to have a debilitating effect.

The economic impact of crises such as the pandemic and bushfires before also lead to multiple social and personal impacts. Modeling using Australian data has estimated that the COVID-19 shutdown is likely to be linked to a future spike of between 750 and 1500 suicide deaths annually associated with the impact of job loss, financial stress and social isolation (Australian Medical Association, 2020). Peterman and colleagues (2020) have documented how economic insecurity, social isolation, reduced health service access and inability to escape violent perpetrators are key pathways through which violence against women may increase during this ongoing crisis period, a situation which may be life-threatening for people locked in homes with violent perpetrators (Molyneaux et al., 2020).

High-risk population groups during the COVID-19 outbreak and response

There has been a global focus on those most at risk of the COVID-19 pandemic with public health measures especially targeted at those who are older adults or have compromised immune systems. When considering mental health it is also important to consider those most at risk of adverse mental health outcomes. For example, people who were adversely impacted by the bushfires, floods or drought may be at a heightened risk for difficulty in coping with the pandemic. People who have a preexisting mental health condition may also experience an increase in symptoms. Australia's First Nations Peoples living in rural communities have also been highlighted as a particularly vulnerable group (Department of Health, 2020) because of the preexisting differences in the health status of this group and reduced access to health care. In order to protect Indigenous communities, the government ordered a lockdown of rural communities in an attempt to keep the virus out.

Another vulnerable population in Australia whose suffering has become almost invisible to the Australian community are people from refugee backgrounds. Asylum seekers in particular are subjected to harsh immigration procedures including immigration detention and temporary visas, leaving them in ongoing situations of uncertainty which have been demonstrated to adversely impact mental health outcomes (Steel et al., 2011). Asylum seekers who have been brought to the Australian mainland from offshore detention for medical treatment are now being held in crowded conditions in hotel accommodation with no opportunities for physical distancing—despite the fact that they already have health problems that put them at greater risk of complications (Burridge, 2020). The Australian government's financial aid package to support people through the COVID-19 crisis has excluded refugees on temporary visas and asylum seekers (Asylum Seeker Resource Centre, 2020) placing a highly vulnerable population at further risk. These exclusions have also applied to the large number of international student and migrant workers in Australia leaving many facing potential destitution with loss of work due to economic shut down and no access to a social safety net.

Both First Nations Peoples and those from refugee backgrounds likely have experienced past traumas which impact on their wellbeing. Situations of lockdown may remind people of conflict conditions which similarly required them to remain inside, such as restrictions placed on the movement of First Nations Peoples until relatively recently, siege situations in Syria, or bombing campaigns in Iraq. These situations can trigger trauma reactions which may be difficult to address in crowded living conditions. Language and cultural differences may make accessing health and support services more challenging for people from cultural and linguistically diverse communities (Refugee Council of Australia, 2019). This can seriously endanger people's lives.

Frontline health workers have been the immediate bulwark against the virus with that group facing one of the highest levels of adverse and potentially fatal COVID-19 outcomes globally. The sense of threat amongst front line workers has only been compounded by national and global shortages in personal protective equipment (PPE) which are essential to supporting health workers working with COVID-19 infected patients. While shortages of PPE were evident in Australia the effectiveness of the public health measures prevented this from emerging as a health disaster, but rather served as a national wake up call. The focus in Australia quickly shifted to the effectiveness of public health control measures being implemented. The inevitable occurrence of mistakes or errors in judgment that will occur in real time implementation of plans with limited information has come under intense public media scrutiny. This has placed extreme pressure on individual health staff who have been subject to extraordinary levels of public and media outrage and criticism following adverse events.

Mental Health Care Infrastructure and COVID-19 response

As with many countries, the mental health system in Australia is struggling with high levels of patient acuity and an under-funded public sector. The need for increased mental health services had been identified as a major policy challenge facing the country (Australian Medical Association, 2018). Although the Australian government has allocated an additional $74 million to mental health care due to the COVID-19 crisis (Morrison, 2020), the substantial uptake of these funds during the first wave of the pandemic is unlikely to address the longer-term mental health need that will present in the years following a pandemic which is when the full burden will most likely manifest (Mak et al., 2009). A potential benefit arising from the COVID-19 crisis has been the need to rapidly to shift the model of mental health care to one that fully integrated Telehealth services with new funding category supporting this model. This shift in ways of providing care may create a greater flexibility and capacity within the mental health service system to provide services to population groups that have previously been excluded from regular access to mental health services due to remoteness or other factors preventing access.

Getting on the front foot with mental health and COVID-19

While there is clear evidence of heighted population concern and psychological distress in Australia these reactions may best be understood and addressed drawing on and promoting models of resilience, grief recovery, posttraumatic growth, hope, and self-compassion as pathways for navigating the current challenges. A key protective factor during times of hardship is resilience, defined as the ability to maintain a sense of equilibrium during and following on from times of adversity (Bonanno, 2004). O'Leary and Ickovics (1995) described three responses to stressors termed survival, recovery, and thriving. Survival refers to continued functioning at an impaired level and implies minimal proactive engagement in daily living. Recovery is the return to previous levels of baseline psychosocial functioning following decline in response to a stressor. Going beyond this baseline is referred to as thriving, a transformational flourishing response borne primarily from changes in cognitive shifts to the challenge presented. Other scholars refer to this transformational positive change as posttraumatic growth (Tedeschi et al., 2018).

Thriving and posttraumatic growth are likely not the first concepts that come to mind as COVID-19 is navigated at individual, family, community, and nation-wide levels. Resilience and coping will come in many forms as we strive for a sense of equilibrium in an ever-changing landscape. Tedeschi and Calhoun (1996) outline five main factors that are indicative of growth following exposure to stressors: relating to others, new possibilities, personal strength, spiritual change, and appreciation of life. Actionable tasks that may support growth include an increased willingness to express emotions and invest in healthy relationships, pursuance of new interests and opportunities, and expressing appreciation for one's strengths and life through gratitude journaling

According to the models of thriving (O'Leary & Ickovics, 1995) and posttraumatic growth (Tedeschi et al., 2018), challenges such as those presented by COVID-19 provide change opportunities through reflection on, and re-assessment of one's self and roles both privately and socially. This may include altered role acquisition (e.g., the child becoming the carer for a parent), role loss (e.g., termination from work), or priority reorganization (e.g., placing greater emphasis on maintaining social connections rather than career building). Perception of the profound stressor may also play a role in the thriving response due to cognitive factors such as self-appraisal and assessment of risk to self, which will influence expectancy outcomes and perceived self-efficacy.

O'Leary (1998) extended the model of thriving to the community level by drawing on Bandura's (1997) concept of *collective efficacy*: a group's beliefs about its organizational abilities to take a course of action leading to successful attainment of outcomes that underpin social thriving. We have seen this in action via community groups such as mutual aid that enable members to be of service to one another while each person maintains a sense of agency by participating within their capacity. The ability to be of service within these groups may serve to behaviorally challenge maladaptive cognitions by providing a sense of contribution, connection, and efficacy. By enabling donors to be of assistance within their personal means and limits, community groups may serve as an avenue for the generation of resilience, thriving and posttraumatic growth, while also providing direct benefit to recipients.

Taking a compassionate stance that limits judgment of self or others as we move through unchartered territories may help us draw on a spirit of kindness as kindred travelers on a shared, unchartered journey. By deliberately drawing on coping strategies that enhance resilience we can not only survive and recover from this devastating virus, but perhaps also grow in the face of adversity. Increasing hopefulness during this difficult time is essential for wellbeing. Hope theory addresses the importance of goals that are achievable within set timeframes in order to increase agency and therefore motivation (Snyder, 2000). Depending on the circumstances, resilience through hope may involve tasks of survival and recovery such as taking a shower, cooking a meal, or attending to a work project. In the thriving phase, a goal such as learning a new skill or taking on a mentally taxing task might be pursued. However, COVID-19 has forced us to slow down and adjust our way of living. Self-compassion entailing kindness to self, acknowledgment that our experiences are common to humanity, and the ability to mindfully observe difficult thoughts and feelings at a distance that precludes over-identification with them (Neff, 2003), may help us to adapt by ensuring we set realistic goals and expectations for ourselves and others.

In the wake of quarantine enforcements due to COVID-19, organizations flooded our inboxes with emails containing self-help information and online courses. However, the plethora of information may be best utilized when placed within the context of sound psychological principles. For example, the unknown trajectory of the virus and the subsequent ongoing changes at the macro level may leave individuals feeling helpless, powerless, and with little sense of control, thereby fostering depressive and anxious symptoms. Therefore, cultivating an internal locus of control may be of benefit. This involves identifying areas of most and least control, and shifting focus and behavior to acting on those things most within our control.

Understanding this paradigm may then help with increasing adherence to practical tasks including good sleep hygiene, healthy eating, exercise, meditation, and spending time outdoors.

One important determinant of mental health particularly relevant during the COVID-19 pandemic is physical activity, with a rapidly increasing body of research documenting the multidirectional relationship between physical activity, physical health and mental health. The anti-depressive and anxiolytic benefits of physical activity for both clinical (Schuch et al., 2019) and non-clinical populations (Rebar et al., 2015) has been well established. Experimental research from healthy volunteers for instance shows that inducing sedentary behavior in healthy people increases levels of depression after 7-days (Edwards & Loprinzi, 2016). Promoting physical activity may also provide an opportunity to promote social connectedness to potentially help alleviate symptoms of psychological distress and improve quality of life. Online technologies including social media platforms offer a novel method of reaching people, particularly during periods of social isolation where face-to-face interventions are prohibited, with preliminary data demonstrating such interventions are acceptable strategies to increase physical activity levels (McKeon et al., 2019). Use of physical activity to support the wellbeing of health workers should be pivotal in introducing wholistic models of mental health care.

Frontline workers are known to have a significant mental health burden during pandemics (Brooks et al., 2018). Data from the Nurses Health cohort study shows that decreases in physical activity over time, are associated with the number of posttraumatic stress symptoms, with higher number of symptoms associated with a steeper decline in physical activity levels (Winning et al., 2017). This is particularly pertinent for healthcare workers on the frontline, and suggests that cases of poor mental health within this workforce may be prevented through, or mitigated through, a focus on "lifestyle psychiatry," and modifiable lifestyle factors including physical activity, diet, smoking and sleep behavior.

It is now the 4th of June, 2020. In the past 2 weeks restrictions in Australia have eased; children are back at school; people are returning to work as required; small gatherings are permitted; some professional team sport is being played, albeit to empty stadiums. Physical distancing remains in place; state and national borders remain closed and we wonder what is coming next. Will there be a second wave? Will it be worse than the first? Bushfire season will soon approach with no chance to process the disaster earlier this year. At a personal level, many of us wonder if we will we continue to have jobs? The authors all work in the tertiary sector; the repercussions for this sector of the pandemic will continue for years. There has been a collapse of the international student sector leaving huge holes in University budgets across the country. We remain optimistic and hope that lessons can be learned from this experience. We know many people are hurting in a variety of ways through isolation, economic, physical, and emotional challenges. However, if academic and creative literature tells us anything, it is that adversity can also lead to adaptation and new possibilities.

Acknowledgement

The authors thank the other members of the Australasian Society for Traumatic Stress Studies Management Committee for discussion and encouraging us to write this piece.

References

Asylum Seeker Resource Centre. (2020). *The ASRC submits petition to Parliament while people seeking asylum lose employment without any COVID-19 safety nets.* https://www.asrc.org.au/2020/04/08/the-asrc-submits-petition-to-parliament-while-people-seeking-asylum-lose-employment-without-any-covid-19-safety-nets/

Australian Bureau of Statistics. (2020). *Household Impacts of COVID-19 Survey.* (4940.0). Australian Bureau of Statistics. https://www.abs.gov.au/AUSSTATS/abs@.nsf/DetailsPage/4940.01-6%20Apr%202020?OpenDocument

Australian Medical Association. (2018). "AMA position statement: Mental health." Retrieved from https://ama.com.au/system/tdf/documents/Mental-Health-2018-%20Position-Statement.pdf?file=1&type=node&id=47704

Australian Medical Association, Brain and Mind Centre, & Orygen Centre for Youth Mental Health (2020). *Covid-19 impact likely to lead to increased rates of suicide and mental illness* [Press release]. https://ama.com.au/media/joint-statement-covid-19-impact-likely-lead-increased-rates-suicide-and-mental-illness

Bandura, A. (1997). *Self-efficacy: The exercise of control.* W.H. Freeman.

Bonanno, G. A. (2004). Loss, trauma, and human resilience: Have we underestimated the human capacity to thrive after extremely aversive events? *The American Psychologist, 59*(1), 20–28. https://doi.org/10.1037/0003-066X.59.1.20

Borchers Arriagada, N., Palmer, A. J., Bowman, D., Morgan, G., Jalaludin, B., & Johnston, F. (2020). Unprecedented smoke-related health burden associated with the 2019–20 bushfires in eastern Australia. *Medical Journal of Australia.* https://www.mja.com.au/journal/2020/213/6/unprecedented-smoke-related-health-burden-associated-2019-20-bushfires-eastern https://doi.org/10.5694/mja2.50545

Brooks, S. K., Dunn, R., Amlôt, R., Rubin, G. J., & Greenberg, N. (2018). A systematic, thematic review of social and occupational factors associated with psychological outcomes in healthcare employees during an infectious disease outbreak. *Journal of occupational and environmental medicine, 60*(3), 248–257.

Burridge, A. (2020). Hotels are no 'luxury' place to detain people seeking asylum in Australia. *The Conversation.* https://theconversation.com/hotels-are-no-luxury-place-to-detain-people-seeking-asylum-in-australia-134544

Centre for Disaster Philanthropy. (2020). 2019–2020 Australian Bushfires. https://disasterphilanthropy.org/disaster/2019-australian-wildfires/

Department of Health: Australian Government. (2020). Coronavirus (COVID-19) advice for Aboriginal and Torres Strait Islander peoples and remote communities. https://www.health.gov.au/news/health-alerts/novel-coronavirus-2019-ncov-health-alert/advice-for-people-at-risk-of-coronavirus-covid-19/coronavirus-covid-19-advice-for-aboriginal-and-torres-strait-islander-peoples-and-remote-communities

Dickman, C. (2020). *Billion animals Uni Sydney.* https://www.sydney.edu.au/news-opinion/news/2020/01/08/australian-bushfires-more-than-one-billion-animals-impacted.html

Edwards, M. K., & Loprinzi, P. D. (2016). Effects of a sedentary behavior–inducing randomized controlled intervention on depression and mood profile in active young adults. *Mayo Clinic Proceedings, 91*(8), 984–998. https://doi.org/10.1016/j.mayocp.2016.03.021

Lifeline (2020). *COVID-19 Impact activates first national emergency appeal in lifeline's 57 year history* [Press release]. https://www.lifeline.org.au/static/uploads/files/20200409-media-release-covid-impacts-activate-lifelines-first-ever-emergency-app.pdf

Mak, I. W. C., Chu, C. M., Pan, P. C., Yiu, M. G. C., & Chan, V. L. (2009). Long-term psychiatric morbidities among SARS survivors. *General hospital psychiatry, 31*(4), 318–326.

McKeon, G., Steel, Z., Wells, R., Newby, J. M., Hadzi-Pavlovic, D., Vancampfort, D., & Rosenbaum, S. (2019). Mental health informed physical activity for first responders and their support partner: A protocol for a stepped-wedge evaluation of an online, codesigned intervention. *BMJ Open, 9*(9), e030668. https://doi.org/10.1136/bmjopen-2019-030668

Molyneaux, R., Gibbs, L., Bryant, R. A., Humphreys, C., Hegarty, K., Kellett, C., Gallagher, H. C., Block, K., Harms, L., Richardson, J. F., Alkemade, N., & Forbes, D. (2020). Interpersonal violence and mental health outcomes following disaster. *BJPsych Open, 6*(1). https://doi.org/10.1192/bjo.2019.82

Morrison, S. (2020). "$1.1 billion to support more mental health, Medicare and domestic violence services." [Press Release.] Retrieved from https://www.pm.gov.au/media/11-billion-support-more-mental-health-medicare-and-domestic-violence-services-0

Murphy, K., & Karp, P. (2020). Borders closing. *The Guardian.* https://www.theguardian.com/world/2020/mar/19/australian-government-moves-to-close-borders-as-new-coronavirus-cases-continue-to-rise

Neff, K. D. (2003). Self-compassion: An alternative conceptualization of a healthy attitude toward oneself. *Self and Identity, 2*(2), 85–101. https://doi.org/10.1080/15298860309032

O'Leary, V. E. (1998). Strength in the face of adversity: Individual and social thriving. *Journal of Social Issues, 54*, 425–446. https://doi.org/10.1111/j.1540-4560.1998.tb01228.x

O'Leary, V. E., & Ickovics, J. R. (1995). Resilience and thriving in response to challenge: An opportunity for a paradigm shift in women's health. *Women's. Health: Research on Gender, Behavior, and Policy, 1*, 121–142.

Peterman, A., Potts, A., O'Donnell, M., Thompson, K., Shah, N., Oertelt-Prigione, S., & van Gelder, N. (2020). *Pandemics and violence against women and children.* https://www.cgdev.org/publication/pandemics-and-violence-against-women-and-children

Rebar, A., Stanton, R., Geard, D., Short, C., Duncan, M., & Vandelanotte, C. (2015). A Meta-Meta-Analysis of the effect of physical activity on depression and anxiety in non-clinical adult populations. *Health Psychology Review, 9*(3), 366–378. https://doi.org/10.1080/17437199.2015.1022901

Refugee Council of Australia. (2019). *Barriers and exclusions: The support needs of newly arrived refugees with a disability.* https://www.refugeecouncil.org.au/disability-report/

Schuch, F., Stubbs, B., Meyer, J., Heissel, A., Zech, P., Vancampfort, D., Rosenbaum, S., Deenik, J., Firth, J., Ward, P., Carvalho, A., & Hiles, S. (2019). Physical activity protects from incident anxiety: A meta-analysis of prospective cohort studies. *Depression and Anxiety, 36*(9), 846–858. https://doi.org/10.1002/da.22915

Snyder, C. R. (2000). Hypothesis: There is hope. In C. R. Snyder (Ed.), *Handbook of hope: Theory, measures, and applications* (pp. 3–21). Academic Press.

Steel, Z. (2020). When the smoke clears: Supporting communitiies after a disaster. *Medicine Today, 21*(3), 10–19. https://medicinetoday.com.au/2020/march/feature-article/when-smoke-clears-supporting-communities-after-disaster

Steel, Z., Momartin, S., Silove, D., Coello, M., Aroche, J., & Tay, K. W. (2011). Two year psychosocial and mental health outcomes for refugees subjected to restrictive or supportive immigration policies. *Social Science & Medicine (1982), 72*(7), 1149–1156. https://doi.org/10.1016/j.socscimed.2011.02.007

Tedeschi, R. G., & Calhoun, L. G. (1996). The Posttraumatic Growth Inventory: Measuring the positive legacy of trauma. *Journal of Traumatic Stress, 9*(3), 455–471. https://doi.org/10.1002/jts.2490090305

Tedeschi, R. G., Shakespeare-Finch, J., Taku, K., & Calhoun, L. G. (2018). *Posttraumatic growth: Theory, research and applications.* Routledge.

Wheaton, M. G., Abramowitz, J., Berman, N., Fabricant, L., & Olatunji, B. (2012). Psychological predictors of anxiety in response to the H1N1 (swine flu) pandemic. *Cognitive Therapy and Research, 36*(3), 210–218. https://doi.org/10.1007/s10608-011-9353-3

Winning, A., Gilsanz, P., Koenen, K. C., Roberts, A. L., Chen, Q., Sumner, J. A., Rimm, E. B., Maria Glymour, M., & Kubzansky, L. D. (2017). Post-traumatic stress disorder and 20-year physical activity trends among women. *American Journal of Preventive Medicine, 52*(6), 753–760. https://www.ajpmonline.org/article/S0749-3797(17)30105-8/fulltext

World Health Organization (WHO). (2018). *International classification of diseases for mortality and morbidity statistics* (11th Revision). https://icd.who.int/browse11/l-m/en

The Future That Awaits Us

Peter Joseph Gloviczki

ABSTRACT
In this autoethnographic exploration, I consider the ongoing social interruption of the COVID 19 pandemic and work to imagine the post-pandemic future that awaits us. I especially employ the autoethnographic tradition to contextualize everyday experiences during these unprecedented times.

On this early summer Sunday, I am up early, having already done pushups and treadmill. I appreciate the invitation to start the morning with movement. I have learned it as the best time for me to workout. Routines can be constricting, no doubt, but this one feels liberating, as in the light behind an open door. Rising amidst our pandemic moment has come to feel similar with each awakening. Though I am good at patterns, even take comfort in them, the banal everyday can be exhausting. In a phone call to a friend yesterday, I wondered about what home means, when I cannot easily leave it, or move as freely as I would like. In such moments, the schedule of movement, the morning routine, takes on added significance. In another context, Jarod Rosello asks: "What was I mourning, what was I grieving for?" (2017, p. 249). I write not to mourn or grieve but to recognize and celebrate the four walls of the home that are keeping me safe.

In the same breath, there is something that has been lost, though: the everyday of social interaction is spinning out. Face to Face now means something more like Platform to Platform, at least for this blip of time in our life on earth. I wonder: is this what Derrida meant when he cautioned: "But within structure there is not only form, relation and configuration. There is also interdependency and a totality which is always concrete" (1978, p. 5). I zoom in on interdependency in that passage, probably misunderstanding it but questioning all the same what social interaction looks like without another to interact with in person. Or at least without the level of in-person interaction we have become accustomed to. We make due, because what else can we do? And we wait in a sacrifice of sorts, but there is a lot to celebrate: the reality of health and healthfulness feels more present. I hear autoethnographer Larry Russell's wise words in my mind: "This is a story about the blessings of age" (2003, p. 225). The message resonates within me. How fortunate I am to be here this morning. I scan the body and again: the weight of breathing in and out takes on that certain pleasure.

If, as it has for me, the COVID 19 pandemic has also encouraged others to look inward, allow me to affirm that response, validate it and make enough space for each of us. Autoethnographers have taught me to find value in the everyday, whatever it might bring. And amidst our ongoing social interruption, I am working on doing that. The work of putting things on pause, of not broadcasting, does not mean I (or we) lack feeling or cease to experience the world as it is. As autoethnographer Erica Hollander writes so beautifully about grief: "It is with me always but I do not always show it to others" (2004, p. 202). Progressing in our lives carries within it the opportunity to rethink who we wish to be post-pandemic. For the physical and emotional work associated with doing that, the eventual reveal may well be worth it. In a hopefully not too distant moment, I imagine a morning where I wake up and workout, as I did this morning. I then go to work, teach my classes and meet friends in person afterward. We eat together and tell stories. We decide, after dessert, to take in a movie. Facing COVID 19, we must prioritize our health and safety. And we do not yet know the future that awaits us, but if it looks something like that, it might be alright. And we might emerge more mindful of the opportunities and challenges that face us.

References

Derrida, J. (1978). *Writing and difference* (Alan Bass, trans.). University of Chicago Press.

Hollander, E. M. (2004). Am I all Right? *Journal of Loss & Trauma*, *9*(3), 201–204. https://doi.org/10.1080/1532502049045589

Rosello, J. (2017). How we endure: Writing, drawing and remembering. *International Review of Qualitative Research*, *10*(3), 242–251.

Russell, L. (2003). Stopping by a cemetery on a snowy morning. *Journal of Loss and Trauma*, *8*(4), 221–227. https://doi.org/10.1080/15325020305880

Index

Note: Figures are indicated by *italics*. Tables are indicated by **bold**. Endnotes are indicated by the page number followed by 'n' and the endnote number e.g., 20n1 refers to endnote 1 on page 20.